Healthy Sun

Healing with Sunshine
And the Myths About Skin Cancer

By Case Adams, Naturopath

Healthy Sun: Healing with Sunshine and the Myths About Skin
Cancer
Copyright © 2010, 2012, 2014 Case Adams
LOGICAL BOOKS
Wilmington, Delaware
http://www.logicalbooks.org
All rights reserved.
Printed in USA
Front cover photo: Oleksandr Kalyna
Back cover image: Roksana Bashyrova

Publishers Cataloging in Publication Data
Adams, Case
Healthy Sun: Healing with Sunshine and the Myths About Skin
Cancer
First Edition
1. Health. 2. Medicine
    Bibliography and References; Index

Library of Congress Control Number: 2009932603

ISBN Paperback: 978-0-9816045-8-9
ISBN ebook: 978-1-936251-06-3

Table of Contents

Introduction

For many, the sun is a mortal enemy. Many of us see the sun only giving us cancer and dry, wrinkled skin. This is added to dehydration, heat exhaustion, drought, solar storm activity and so many other environmental problems blamed on the sun.

Is the sun really our enemy?

If the sun were our enemy, how is it that humanity and uncountable other creatures have thrived for millions of years under the sun? How is it that early humans spent predominantly all day outside in the sun? How is it that civilizations living in arid lands with little rain and abundant sunshine thrived for centuries? Why were they not killed off by the sun? Why did they not all die from skin cancer – especially without any sunscreen!

Here we will show that the sun is hardly our enemy. The sun, in fact, is a giver of life. The sun is our primary source of heat. Directly and indirectly, it is our primary means for nutrition. The sun stimulates many biochemicals required to maintain health and cognition. The sun rises each day with periodicity and rhythm, entraining our metabolic functions to flow with consistency.

The sun is our friend: As long as we use it with care, respect and wisdom.

The information presented here is a blend of ancient science and modern research. The ancients were no dummies. They were as intelligent – if not more – than we are. No, they did not create some of the technologies we have. They were not able to peer as deeply into space. They were not able to see tiny bacteria, living cells or DNA molecules.

They also did not create an industrial complex complete with toxic wastes and emissions that risk life on this planet.

The ancients also spent significantly more time outside, within nature. The ancients, by necessity, had to work and synchronize with the elements of nature. This means they had more time to study and connect with nature's rhythms. They had to utilize the elements like the sun and the stars for survival and navigation. They had to understand the relationship between their bodies and the elements. Quite simply, they were the experts when it comes to living with the sun.

Practically every ancient society revered the sun. Middle East petroglyphs from the Neolithic era illustrated the sun as a personality who traveled in a large boat or ship. This vision of a sun demigod was passed on through many generations. The Egyptians recognized the sun as Ra, and constructed a gigantic boat to symbolize his vehicular motion through the sky. This 2500 B.C. *Khufu* boat, housed in the Great Pyramid of Giza, was over 125 feet long.

This vision of the sun demigod driving a chariot was also held among other ancient cultures. The Japanese described the sun as *Amarterasu;* the Romans as *Sol Invictus;* the Greeks as *Helios;* the Nordics as *Sol;* and the ancient Kizil caves from the Kucha region of China depict a sun-demigod wearing a crown and armor while seated with ankles crossed on a two-seated chariot.

The ancient peoples of Himalaya and the Indus Valley envisioned the sun as a personality as well. They saw the sun as a great demigod who traveled by chariot through the heavens on a periodic basis. The Vedic texts referred to the sun-demigod as *Viviswan* or *Surya. Surya* was seen as a powerful personality who was devoted to God. The texts of the *Rg-Veda* describe Surya as dedicated to providing a clear passageway for God's light.

The ancient tribes of Israel recognized the personality of the sun as *Shamshoun,* which is translated to "God's servant." It is thought that *Samson* from the *Book of Judges* details some of the life and times of Samson. This discussion also connects particular activities, such as standing between two posts during the dawn and two pillars at dusk. It is also suspicious that the Samson narrative takes 12 chapters, which may have symbolized the 12 months and/or 12 zodiac houses. Samson was also considered a devoted servant of God.

The ancient French culture of the Basque also saw the sun as a personality, named *Eguzki.* Eguzki was also seen as a great saint and protector. They believed that the sun brightened the sky as part of its protection of the earth and its inhabitants.

Cenncroithi was the name of the Irish sun-demigod, revered prior to the coming of the Christians. Cenncroithi was ceremoniously respected during the solstice periods.

The Romans named the sun's deity *Sol,* which also translates to 'sun' and is the root of 'solar.' The *Sol Indiges* and *Sol Invictus* were also applied in the worship of *Sol,* and this carried on through the time of Constantine. The pagan solstice ceremony was often held on December 25, which irritated the early Church. The Church decided that the ceremonial birth of Jesus ought to be held on that day to dissuade the worship of the sun. As a result, we now have Christmas on the same day of an ancient ceremony for the sun.

The Sumerians of Mesopotamia from 2000 B.C. revered the sun-demigod as *Utu*. Consistent with the Greeks, Aryans, Romans and many others, Utu was a demigod among a range of other demigods, while *Anu* was worshiped as the King of the demigods – God. Also similar to the role played in other cultures, Utu was related with the moon demigod *Nanna* and the demigod governing the weather, *Ishkur*.

The Uratu tribe of the Asia Minor region during the 9th through 6th centuries B.C. also revered the sun as a demigod, named *Artinis* or *Shivini*. Shivini/Artinis was seen as one of the three principle demigods, and was envisioned as holding up the power of the sun while kneeling. The other two principle gods were *Theispas*, who governed thunder, and the Supreme God, *Khaldi*, who was considered the God of the gods. Shivini/Artinis again is seen as a devoted servant of this God of gods.

Among the Slavs of northern Europe, we find similar descriptions of the sun. *Svarog* or *Dabog* was revered as the demigod of the sun, who also governed fire, while *Rod* was considered the Creator of Svarog. The Slavs also recognized a trilogy of principle demigods, called *Triglav*. This trilogy was seen as composed of *Veles, Svarog,* and *Rod* – with some variation on the particular names, as many Slav tribes had different names for the same diety.

The Pawnee Indians of North America were one of many North American Indian tribes that revered the sun-demigod. The Pawnees called the sun *Shakuru*. Shakuru was part of an assembly of deities that organized the sky from east (masculine) to west (feminine). These dieties were envisioned to have taken birth from a principle God called *Tirawa*. Tirawa brought together the stars, the moon, the sun, the weather, east and west, and all the other elements. Strict Pawnee ceremonies continued until the end of the nineteenth century.

The Ossetian peoples of the Northern Caucasus region now known as Eastern Russia revered a similar array of demigods. The sun-demigod was known as *Wasterzhi*, and the principle God of the demigods was known as *Xwycau*. A number of other demigods, similar to other cultures were also revered among the Ossetians, and their demigods were referenced among various Christian saints.

The Mayans of Central America also revered this council structure of demigods. The personalities who represented the various elements were led by the significant leader and supreme Deity, *Quetzalcoatl*. The sun was seen as a demigod who came into being through a transformation of the *Popol Vuh* among the Supreme and His wife. This gave birth to the sun and moon. The sun demigod's name as translated from Mayan texts is *Kinich Ahau*, and he was seen as having features similar to a jaguar.

In the Bronze Age, Nordic cultures of 1500 B.C.E. also documented a personal representation of the sun riding upon a chariot being pulled by a horse. *Sol* was his name, and *Sunna* was his goddess. Incidentally, the spoked wheel technology of *Sol's* chariot wheels appears to predate the invention of spoked wheels among the Nords and any other culture by many centuries.

A few thousand years later, Saint Francis of Assisi referred respectfully to "brother sun," respecting the sun as a fellow servant and provider of God's light. In his famous hymn the *Cantical of the Sun* (1224), St. Francis wrote:

"Be praised my Lord, through all Your creatures, especially through my lord brother sun, who brings the day; and gives Your light through him. And he is beautiful and radiant in all his splendor! Of You, Most High, he bears the likeness."

Throughout the centuries, the sun has also been seen as a critical component of nature's elements. Indeed, many ancient texts described the universe as stratified with layers of elements. The Greeks and the Egyptians also subscribed to the concept of elemental stratification. The Chinese texts of the Emperors, the ancient Vedic texts, the Greeks, the Arabians, and the technologies of many other ancient cultures were firmly entrenched in this understanding of an elemental layering of matter.

The ancient elemental view of the world eventually influenced the sciences of chemistry, biology, and physics as taught throughout Europe and the Mediterranean of the middle ages through the Renaissance. Today, modern western science assumes this stratification of elements in the form of solids, liquids, gasses and so on.

These of course are now fundamental to our understandings in molecular matter, earth sciences, space, physiology, and biology.

Similar elemental derivatives also played a key role in the Egyptian, North American Indian, Japanese, Mayan, and Polynesian cultures. In the North American Indian tradition, for example, the elements of nature are related as 'brother sun,' 'mother earth,' 'grandmother moon,' the 'four brothers of the wind,' and the 'four directions.' The Japanese *godai*, meaning 'five great,' also reflects the physical elements, namely *chi* (earth), *sui* (water), *kaze* (wind), *ka* (fire) and ku (sky or void). A similar five-element vision was also embraced by the ancient Chinese and Vedic cultures, along with others. The Greeks utilized a four corner 'Hellenic' model of air, fire, earth and water. Modern western science has inherited a similar stratification of elements. In western science terms, 'earth' relates to solids, 'water' relates to liquids, 'fire' or 'sun' relates to thermal radiation, 'wind' or 'air' relates to gases, while 'space,' 'metal,' 'void' or 'sky' relates to the realm of the electromagnetic.

Around 3,000 B.C.E., peoples of the English isles erected what is now thought to be a large calendar and timepiece called *Stonehenge*. Most consider this structure to have provided a platform for some sort of religious ceremony. At the very least, its ghostly granite pillars tell of an ancient focus upon the sun and skies. Its remote location and stone reveal a mysterious technology used to transport the stones. These indicate the existence of a mysterious culture with a tremendous focus upon the sun's motions and effects. The arrangements of the stones and pillars display an orientation for aligning the winter's and summer's solstice periods, lining up sunrises and sunsets with the position of area landmarks. This indicates a sophistication tied to the mechanics and positioning of the sun. The advanced format of the alignments between the pillars and surrounding area suggests a rigorous methodology and science surrounding the purpose of the structure.

The circa 3500 B.C.E. *Knowth* tomb from Ireland offers an even earlier synchronization mechanism with the sun, with a passageway that traced the sun's journey through the sky. As with early Egyptian, Indus Valley and Babylonian architectural structures that coordinated the sun's path through different types of chambers, the tomb illustrated a desire to coordinate the path of the sun with the passage of time and endeavor.

Sundials of many forms were the norm in these ancient cultures. Some were table-sized flat surfaces with needles, while others were more complex. Concaved discs, called hemicycliums, created a bowl shape. This shape corrects slight variances related to seasonal changes. Round discs were also typical, illustrating not only the passing of the sun but the approximate day and year in relation to the equinox. The *Jantar Mantar* of the Indus region was an ancient architectural building developed to form what is called the equinoctial dial. This building had an angular side that reflected the path of the sun through the sky along with its declination to the horizon and constellations. This allowed the viewer to predict future positions of planets, sun, moon and other stars. The *Jantar* was also a *yantra* – a symbolic representation of a higher realm within the universe.

Almost every ancient culture, including the Indian, Chinese, Egyptian, Greek, Roman, Mayan, Polynesian, Aboriginal and others, developed instruments to measure the sun, moon and planets' relative motion through the sky. Recordings of sun and star positions have been discovered in hieroglyphs from ancient Babylon dating back to 4200 B.C.E. and the Sumerians of 4000 B.C.E. Archeological findings dating between 600 and 1300 B.C.E. credited to the Assyrians illustrated sun and star maps against the backdrop of eighteen constellations. The constellations or houses served as references for the movement and positioning of the sun, moon and stars. By 600 B.C.E., the Greeks and Arabians had shrunk the number of constellations or zodiac locations down to twelve – consistent with the earlier Vedic version.

Just as our modern scientists endeavor with behavioral studies to understand the connection between our environment and behavior, these ancient researchers endeavored to understand how our behavior relates to the positions of the sun and stars. Those who understood this science were also highly regarded in those societies.

We have thus found curiously sophisticated means of recording the positioning of the sun and moon among many archeological findings. One of these is the ephemeris. The ephemeris measures and records the relative positions of the sun, stars and planets at any particular moment. This geometric tool is thousands of years old and has been used in a number of ancient cultures. It is still in use today.

The ancient *Jyotish Vedanga* of the early Vedic culture documents one of the earliest and most advanced forms of mathematical astrology and astronomy. Some date the original written work at 1400 BCE, while other notable Vedic scholars date its origin thousands of years earlier, at 3000-4000 BCE. The *Jyotisa* formalized a sidereal zodiac, and integrated an ephemeris with the position of the planets and major stars. The ancient *Jyotisa* system calculated the sidereal lunar cycle into a 27-28-day *nakshatra*, with each sidereal day also divided into four quadrants, or *padas*. The total number of *padas* was 108. Each *pada* was connected to the motion and dominance of a principle star. Twelve zodiac houses were defined, and the relative positions of the sun, stars and planets were charted through these twelve houses.

The ancient Chinese culture also used a similar astronomical measurement system. Ancient Chinese astrology dates back to at least the Shang dynasty of some 3600 years ago. The Chinese zodiac was based upon a twelve-year solar cycle, each represented by a particular animal: In order, they consist of the *rat, ox, tiger, rabbit, dragon, snake, horse, ram, monkey, rooster, dog,* and *boar*. As each animal-solar year rotated through the cycles of the five elements (earth, water, fire, metal and wood), a sixty-year cycle was calculated. Twenty-eight total constellations were measured and watched as they traveled through the skies. The Chinese were also known to utilize an ephemeris – the interrelationships of angular positions of the sun, stars and planets. Planets were also associated with the five elements, and their respective positions were said to influence those elements in a particular way.

The focus of many ancient traditions upon the movements and effects of the sun gave rise to a variety of similar yet culturally unique timepieces and calendars. Notable early calendars include the Chinese calendar, the Vedic calendar, the Julian calendar, the Coptic calendar, the Malayalam calendar, the Jalali calendar and many others.

The oldest appears to be the Vedic calendar, derived from measuring the sun's annual path interfaced with the path of the moon's cycles. The year was divided into 27 moons, while each fortnight was divided into two weeks. The days of the week were also related to the celestial sky, with *Ravi*, meaning sun for Sunday, *Soma* or moon for Monday, *Mangala* or Mars for Tuesday, *Budha* or Mercury for Wednesday, *Guru* or Jupiter for Thursday, *Shukra* or Venus for Friday, and *Shani* or Saturn for Saturday.

Though similarities are difficult to ignore, the early Roman and later Julian calendars are significantly different in many ways. The Julian calendar formulates the twelve months with 30-31 days with a leap year alternating February between 28 and 29 days. This of course has been assumed with the current western calendar system.

The geometric and rhythmic motion of the sun with respect to constellations and time gave rise to early mathematics. Mathematical formulas were used by the ancient Egyptians as early as 3000 B.C. Earlier we find mathematical formulae recorded in the texts of the Chinese monarchs of 3500 B.C. They set forth various measurements and calculations on natural relationships, including the periodic motion and angular positions of the sun and stars.

We also find the ancient Vedic texts of 4500 B.C.E. illustrating a mathematical and scientific view of the earth's rhythms. These included calculations of the number of universes, planets, species, and even a description of the atom. These early mathematical revelations came to influence the scientific culture of later cultures with regard to the measurements of sun's motion with respect to time and behavior.

From the earliest of these texts, we find a common acceptance that the physical world synchronizes with a pacing or pulse timed with the sun's motion. As these relationships developed within different cultures, they were passed through the generations via master-student relationships and cross-cultural travels.

The measurement of nature's rhythmic basis was inherited by western science through the ancient Greeks. The famed Greek Pythagoras of the sixth century B.C.E. was considered by many in the West to be instrumental in developing mathematical relationships among the rhythms of nature. Pythagoras and his students combined reason, logic, and learning from previous teachers with the observation of nature. From these they discovered an affinity between the rhythms of nature, the harmony of music, and the mathematical relationships between integers and their ratios. While Pythagoras guided many of those principles directly, credit for many insights presented as Pythagorean concepts was also due to a number of associates and students who learned and taught cooperatively within the renowned Pythagorean community.

Through the works of Philolaus of Tarentum, we learned Pythagoras found that the rhythms of song and instrumentation resonated with the rhythms of the sun and stars. All of these were brought into proportion through mathematical relationships. This same approach led the Pythagoreans to perceive various other connected rhythms within nature. While Pythagoras may or may not be responsible for the famous *Pythagorean Theorem,* he is still considered the "father of numbers." He is also to be credited with the methods of logical reasoning that blossomed later through the teachings of Plato, Aristotle, Socrates, and Ptolemy.

Second century Greek Claudius Ptolemaeus was also known as Ptolemy. Ptolemy was a famed mathematician, astronomer, and natural scientist from Alexandria. He was responsible for a number of treatises that influenced natural scientists over the next 1500 years. His book *Harmonics* focused on the rhythmic qualities of music theory. His *Optics* treatise covered the realms of light rays and vision, and his book *Geography* established many of the principles utilized by geographers and cartographers in mapping and quantifying spatial relationships.

These ancient Greeks proposed that the synergies of nature were all tied to the motions of the sun. This assumption greatly influenced the progression of natural science for many centuries to come. The scientific contributions of Hippocrates, Pythagoras, Socrates, Plato, Aristotle, Copernicus, and others established the groundwork for centuries of progressive scientific endeavor and a reverence for mathematical modeling. The fundamental understanding that the sun and earth moved with a periodic procession stimulated the notion of mathematical relationships within nature, which became the basis for further correlation.

The mathematical calculations necessary to make these associations were significant. Ptolemy documented many of these calculations in a respected scientific treatise on astrology and astronomy. In this groundbreaking work called *Mathematike Syntaxis* –

also known as *Almagest* – Ptolemy recorded many of the mathematical and behavioral relationships used in calculating the relative positions between the earth, sun, stars, planets and constellations. This and other works illustrated how the ephemeris could be used to 'read' human behavior. The *Almagest* was composed of two treatises, one called the *Tetrabiblos* and the other called the *Planetary Hypotheses*. The *Tetrabiblos* focused on the astrological elements, and the *Planetary Hypotheses* focused on a cosmological positioning of the universe. His solar system proposal consisted of a nesting of spherical shells in which the planets moved.

The works of Hipparchus, another early Greek astrologer, were used extensively in Ptolemy's works. Hipparchus was respected as a great mathematician – given credit for the founding of trigonometry. The *Almagest* – like the other works of Ptolemy – was embraced by Arabic, Roman and European natural scientists until the sixteenth century. His calculations used angular geometry and trigonometry extensively, correlating the angles between heavenly bodies with natural occurrences.

Ptolemy's *geocentric* earth-centered view of the universe gradually gave way to the *heliocentric* model proposed by Copernicus, Kepler and Galileo. This of course described the earth as encircling the sun. Though Ptolemy's model was stricken, most of the geometric relationships he described are still recognized and utilized.

An indication of the complexity of Greek solar astronomy was revealed recently with the reconstruction of a two-thousand year old Greek astronomical calculator. Containing an excess of thirty gears, the *Antikythera Calculator* was found by researchers exploring a shipwreck near the island of Antikythera a century ago. The relic had been a mystery since its discovery, as researchers of various disciplines have speculated on its purpose. In 2006, university researchers from Carkiff, Athens, and Thessalonika used x-ray imaging technology to unravel the relic's purpose. They concluded the mechanism – consisting of wheels and dials made of bronze – is effectively the world's oldest computer. A team of researchers from the National Archaeological Museum of Athens was able to reconstruct it. This replica of the relic rotates the sun and each planet's position through the earth's sky – accurately predicting the positioning of the sun, moon and many planets on a given day, revealing its angular relationship with respect to time.

This attunement with nature and a reverence for the sun reflects the reality that our ancestors intently studied, practiced and understood the value of the sun. As we will discuss, this reverence of the sun included using the sun for healing. The ancients knew the sun had medicinal qualities through careful observation and application. They also knew the sun was needed for maintaining ultimate wellness. Thus we find many of the great ancient physicians such as Shen Nong, Huang ti, Amenhotep, Imhotep, Hammurabi, Galen, Hippocrates, Aristotle, Pythagoras, Anaxagoras, Asclepiades, Pliny, Rhazes, Isaac Judaeus, Arnold of Villanova, Hildegard von Bingen and Paracelsus applied sunlight therapeutically. In later years, we find that well-known physicians Thomas Sydenham, Theodor Palm, August Rollier, Arnold Rikli, Hermann Brehmer, Dio Lewis, Niels Finsen, Oskar Bernhard, Benedict Lust, Jethro Kloss, John Harvey Kellogg, Herbert Shelton and Bernard Jensen were all proponents of the use of sunshine in their medical therapies.

Modern humankind has failed miserably when it comes to living with and within nature. Instead of honoring the sun, we have retreated from it – as one might run from a threatening bear. Along the way, we have diverted from our respect for the elements. We have ignored the wisdom of the ancients that taught of a natural world inherent with wisdom, design and consciousness.

As a result, our modern research approaches nature from a diametrically different perspective. Our scientists peer into nature using microscopes and telescopes from sanitary laboratories with an objectivity that separates us from the rhythms and subtle qualities of nature. While having its advantages, this objectivity has unfortunately disconnected us from the practical uses of nature's elements.

Reconnecting with the benefits of sunshine is not difficult, however. Most of us have felt the warmth of the sun's rays seeping through an open window. Most of us have welcomed the diffusion of the light of sunrise in the morning with increased energy and clarity. Most of us have been awestruck by an enchanted sunset. Thus, it will not be difficult to comprehend the implications of the research and information presented here. We are simply too connected to the sun to have forgotten its goodness.

What might prove difficult, however, is reversing the last few decades of media and medical establishment proclamations that the sun is dangerous to our health. We may have a tough time forgetting all the warnings we have received about the sun and its "deadly" nature. For this reason, we have provided a plethora of research illustrating the opposite.

Perhaps the information presented here will help change some of that. Perhaps the research presented here will illustrate that while they may have had good intentions, the researchers and their institutions did not have the entire picture in view when they jumped to the conclusion that the sun causes skin cancer. Like a purloined letter, perhaps our medical establishment's desperate search for effective new medical treatments may just uncover a treatment that is already shining down upon us every day.

Chapter One

The Rhythmic Sun

Every day the sun rises and sets, creating a repetitious cycle. Life on this planet cycles with the sun, adjusting slightly with every variance and nuance. The seasons change as the rotation of the earth varies with respect to its orbit around the sun. Climates are altered with periodic changes in solar storms. These seasonal and climatic variances are reflected in the habits and behavior of every organism on the planet. Most plants wax in the spring and wane in the fall. Birds and other wildlife migrate with this seasonal periodicity. Their travels are synchronized with the seasons and climates, as some seasonally relocate to precisely the same location inhabited the previous year.

The energy of the sun is primarily due to the sun's electromagnetic radiation, hurtling at us at 186,282 miles per second from a heat source estimated to be 93 million miles away.

Scientific analysis has estimated the surface of the sun is about 5,760 degrees Kelvin; yet its corona – or radiance – is estimated to be between 1,000,000 and 5,000,000 degrees Kelvin. The sun's radiance will deposit between 1,000 and 1,300 watts of power onto the earth's surface per square meter. This problem is also referred to as the *coronal heating problem:* Why is the sun's corona so much hotter than its surface? While some propose that the sun's radiation comes from nuclear fusion reactions occurring deep within the sun's core – like many others, this mystery still lies unsolved.

The sun is also magnetic. Its magnetic field fluctuates to up to 3,000 times its normal range. The sun also emits solar flares, which appear to our eyes and instruments to be massive eruptions spewing up to 20 billion tons of matter into space. On a mass basis, researchers estimate the sun represents 99.8 percent of the total mass of this solar system. The planets are quite tiny compared to the sun.

The sun influences the earth's motion, warmth, spin, weather systems, tectonics, magnetism, ocean currents, air circulation, and many other qualities. Without the companion of the sun, the earth would simply not exist as we know it. A delicate balance exists between the sun's electromagnetic rays and the earth's atmosphere. The atmosphere shields and protects life on the planet by absorbing

13

and neutralizing many rays that would likely delete life otherwise. Plants and trees also reduce heat. They absorb ultraviolet rays for photosynthesis and redirect other rays in the form of colors. In the oceans, plankton and various other algae also absorb the sun's rays on the water during photosynthesis.

Plants and animals also create a balance between the atmospheric levels of nitrogen, oxygen and carbon dioxide. As we know now from humanity's interference with the carbon cycle, the unchecked expansion of one group of organisms can create an imbalance that can endanger many other populations.

The respective positions between the sun, earth and moon also influence ocean tidal rhythms, encouraging the exchange of food between ocean organisms and land organisms. The upwelling and down-welling exchanges between deep cold waters with warm tropical waters rotate and recycle the ocean's various biochemicals and marine organisms. These surface water gradients in turn influence wind and weather with their temperature variations.

We see a similar circulation pattern throughout our atmosphere; rotating air temperature, water vapor, and air pressure between the troposphere, stratosphere, mesosphere, thermosphere and ionosphere. These atmospheric layers interact uniquely with the sun's radiation. The stratosphere, for example, contains higher levels of ozone, which absorb ultraviolet-B rays in the 270-315 nanometer (NM) range. Ozone's filtering effects screen over 98% of the sun's ultraviolet-B rays, as well as some far infrared radiation.

Humanity has only recently become aware of the many forms of radiation the sun emits. Outside of ultraviolet rays, the sun produces radio waves, visible light rays, ultraviolet rays, infrared radiation, x-rays, gamma rays, cosmic rays and microwaves. The earth's atmosphere blocks much of the x-rays, cosmic rays, gamma rays and ultraviolet rays – depending upon ozone levels. Meanwhile, a good portion of the sun's visible and infrared radiation is let through. In all it is estimated that the atmosphere blocks about 40% of the sun's total radiation. About half of the heating of the earth's surface is thought to be caused by infrared radiation from the sun. Visible wavelengths also heat the surface. This does not include the thermal heat generated by the earth itself – a significant but difficult to measure source of heat.

On the grand scale, our solar system is only one small solar system among many, revolving around a thermal core of our spiral-shaped Milky Way galaxy. The sun is one of hundreds of billions of stars that encircle our Milky Way galaxy at a speed about 500 miles per second. One revolution of the sun around the center of this galaxy is thought to take about 250 million years. Furthermore, cosmological observations now indicate the Milky Way is but one of hundreds of billions of other galaxies within our observable universe. This universal megacosm consists of a collection of larger and smaller galaxies, each revolving with unique precision within a grander scheme of motion. Like our Milky Way, most galaxies rotate with a predominantly spiral shaped structure: Their spirals uniquely reflect many of the same parameters observed in the oscillations of electromagnetic fields.

Because the sun is tilted about 23.5 degrees from the axis of north and south, it rotates progressively with seasonal changes in magnetism, temperature and light. In June, the northern portion of the planet is tilted towards the sun, giving that part of the planet summertime, warmer temperatures, and longer days. During December, the southern part of the planet is tilted towards the sun, giving that part of the planet warmer temperatures and longer days. Summers on each pole have no nighttime and winters have no daytime. Of course, those winters are extremely cold. The moments when the earth's tilt is at its greatest on each side is called the *solstice*. There are two periodic solstices each year – occurring around June 21 and December 21. This means there are two days each year when daylight and nighttime have equivalent periods: When the sun is at an even angle with the equator. This is called the *equinox*. Like the solstice, the equinox occurs precisely twice a year – in March and September.

The rotation of the earth with its slight tilt and recurring extremes also lends to other earthy periodic movements. From large and small, nature can be measured periodically and rhythmically in relation to the sun's relative position in the sky. One complete season from solstice to solstice is appropriately called one *period* of a cyclic *waveform*. The timing of this period in combination with the amplitude or aspect (23.5 degrees) creates a precise waveform, which when charted over its period of twelve months. This forms one complete *rhythm* of the earth's rotational motion with respect to the sun.

The Human Solar Clock

The sun drives the human body's metabolism in a number of ways. There are four types of basic human cycles: *Circadian (circa*=about; *dian*=a day) – more or less in the range of a day; *Ultradian* – less than a day; *Infradian* – more than a day; and *Circannual* – in the range of a year.

Over the past century, researchers have been vigorously hunting for the source for the body's biological clockworks. In 1929, two Harvard researchers John Fulton and Percival Bailey studied disrupted sleep rhythms among patients with hypothalamus lesions. They concluded a mysterious link between the endocrine system and sleep cycles.

In 1958, Harvard's Dr. Woody Hastings and Dr. Paul Mangelsdorf illustrated how the marine species *G. polyedra* lit up the night's ocean timed to the sun's path. Exposing the tiny plant to various light pulses at different times, Dr. Hastings concluded some internal biological mechanism within the organism must respond to the sun, switching on and off its illuminating appearance. Over the next decade, various other organisms – including humans – were observed maintaining rhythmic biological responses in conjunction with sunlight.

This research began a focused hunt to corner the body's biological connection to light. Researchers assumed that plants and animals possessed cell-switching mechanisms sensitive to light. Controversy took hold in the 1960s when researchers from Germany's Max Planck Institute published a study showing that human biological rhythms were not light-driven as had been suggested. Charles Czeisler, M.D., Ph.D., an eminent Harvard sleep researcher for several decades with over 180 research papers under his belt, questioned that research. Upon visiting the Planck facility, he found that although the subjects' outside lighting was controlled, they were still able to switch on and off indoor lights within their rooms. Apparently, even weak indoor lights can disrupt or entrain the body's clocks. In the years following, numerous light studies done elsewhere confirmed humans' biological clockworks responded to light.

Most human light research has put subjects into caves or other light-controlled dwellings. These dwellings were removed of any cues as to time and place. Multiple studies indicated that the human circadian rhythm was about 25 hours. In 1985, Max Planck's Dr. Rutger Wever monitored temperature cycles, illustrating daily cycles of 21 and 28 hours instead of this 25-hour daily cycle. Furthermore, he found that body core temperatures quickly adjusted to the new light schedules. These studies indicated that the body's circadian cycles, which include the daily cycling of cortisol, melatonin and other hormones and neurotransmitters through the body, appear to be governed by the sun's path.

In 1972, University of Chicago researcher Dr. Robert Moore dropped radioactive label material in rats' eyes and traced its pathway from retinal neurons to two small clusters of neurons deep within the hypothalamus. Two centrally located pinhead-sized clusters of about 10,000 nerve cells called the *suprachiasmatic nuclei* (or SCN cells) were found. The SCN cells were heralded as the biological clock researchers had been looking for over so many decades. Over the next few years, Dr. Moore and his associates traced synaptic contacts with retinal afferent dendrites though the metabolism of young rats to confirm that SCN cells entrained their switching mechanisms to light (Lenn *et al.* 1977).

For the next two decades, Dr. Moore and other researchers, including Dr. Charles Weitz, Dr. David Welsch, and Dr. Eric Herzog, investigated these SCN cells from various aspects. Without synchronized SCN cells, an animal's body rhythms would collapse into chaotic patterns. These SCN cells were observed primarily residing within the hypothalamus. It was assumed that the body's clock was located within the hypothalamus.

These SCN cells appear to connect the hypothalamus with the activities of the pineal gland – a small conical structure lying above the posterior end of the third ventricle. The pineal gland receives impulses directly from the optic nerves. This seemed to confirm that SCN cells were the human body's switching mechanism for a light-driven body clock.

SCN cells are implicated in the secretion of most if not all the major hormones and neurotransmitters within the body. They appear to switch on in response to light pulses as they are received by the pineal gland. The mechanism for this appears to be a double-neuron oscillation guided by a combination of light and genetic expression (Ikonomov *et al.* 1994, Fukada 2002).

As the research on the genetic connection to SCN cell activity unfolded, it became evident that the activities of the thousands of oscillating nerve cells making up the SCN cell region are somehow expressed through a set of clock-oriented genes (Kalsbeek *et al.* 2006). Recent genetic research has identified several clockwork genes. The central CLOCK gene has been identified as 3111T/C; rs1801260 (Benedetti *et al.* 2007) and APRR9 in plants. Other clockwork genes have been identified as BMAL, PER, CRY (cryptochrome-12q23q24.1), and DEC genes (Gomez-Abellan 2007, Kato *et al.* 2006). These genes have been identified through responses to light and measured circadian biowaves.

Early suspicions were raised about the assumption of SCN cells only existing within the hypothalamus. Gradually, *in vitro* and *in vivo* testing demonstrated that various cells throughout the body contain individual SCN cells. In 1973, Yamaoka reported finding SCN cells in the region of the thyroid gland.

Over the next few years, enough dissecting had been done to demonstrate that SCN cells exist throughout the human body. Studies on light inducement have confirmed that these genetically expressed switches around the body respond to light, and exist within the testes, ovaries, kidneys, and most other organs. They have also been found in adipose cells, nerve cells, and cartilage cells.

The work of Dr. H. Okamura (2005) from the Kobe University School of Medicine confirmed that these clock cell genes are located throughout most of the body's major tissue and organ systems. Apparently the genetic expressions of SCN cell oscillations are coupled with the independent clockwork genes in these various locations of the body, and this coupling (or resonating) of genetic expressions synchronizes the pacing of the SCN activities of these cell locations.

Each of the SCN genes is expressed through a unique disposition. The PER expression, for example, is increased by light exposure during the night, yet remains unstimulated by increased light exposure during the day (Shearman *et al.* 1997).

Further research has revealed that these cells are responsive not only to light, but also to selected mRNA and prostaglandin molecules on a concurrent basis. It has become apparent that every cell seems to have its own independent clockworks, and groups of cells synchronize their clocks to a common setting. The genetic structures of the SCN cells have been further investigated, indicating these clockworks have precise genetic switching mechanisms (Buijs *et al.* 2006).

This indicates, quite simply, that the body's various clockworks bridge sunlight with the alignment between the inner physiology and the pacing of metabolism. A variance from this alignment would naturally link to an alteration of metabolism – disease, in other words. Through a combination of *in vitro* elimination and research on animals, a number of studies have confirmed that damage or mutation to these clockwork genes can result in various disease models. For example, damage to the Per1 and Per2 genes has been linked with a number of human cancer models (Chen-Goodspeed and Cheng 2007).

Understandably, the clockwork genes have also been indelibly linked to the rhythmic release of hormones. Clockwork genes are now considered the key regulators (or mediators) for all metabolic processes. Mutations of human clock genes have been linked to metabolic syndrome (Gomez-Abellan *et al.* 2007), bone marrow CD34 immune cell availability (Tsinkalovsky *et al.* 2007), depression (Benedetti *et al.* 2007), and glutathione function (Igarashi *et al.* 2007). Clock genes are disrupted in mania-like behavior (Roybal *et al.* 2007). The clock genes have also been observed mediating expression of the plasminogen activator inhibitor, yielding a greater risk of heart attack (Chong *et al.* 2006). In 2005, researchers from the University of Pittsburgh's School of Medicine found that bipolar disorder was also linked to a disruption of clock genetic expression (Mansour 2005).

The clock genes apparently correlate information from the SCN cells with various peripheral timing cues from around the body. One of the more important synchronizing mechanisms for these genes along with light is feeding schedules. There is an apparent entrainment to feeding cycles and energy metabolism connected with the SCN/CLOCK gene interaction (Mendoza 2007). Alcohol consumption also appears to substantially alter the expression patterns of a large population of clock genes. The PER genes – especially among brain cells – are significantly affected by alcohol consumption (Spanagel *et al.* 2005).

Recent research indicates that the clock genes work by way of a feedback loop using genetic transcription and translation in alternating steps, with protein phosphorylation via kinases reactivating expression loops of the WC-1 and WC-2 proteins. These are apparently switched on and off through the induction of light to heat (Lakin-Thomas 2006). Cry1 seemingly mediates CLOCK/Bmal1 complex repression, which sets up a feedback response (Sato *et al.* 2006). Further research has uncovered the potential of prostaglandin-2 as an activation-switch for resetting these genes, leading researchers to propose a connection between pain and the biological clock. These feedback loops have also been referred to as rhythmic, with a conserved control of gene transcription regulation (Hardin 2004).

It also appears that these SCN neurons are coupled to (or resonate with) other cells. Through a co-signaling process linked to glucocorticoid production, sympathetic nerve activity and other metabolic systems, activation of genetic alterations by SCN are stimulated by sunlight and other waveforms. Organ-based SCN neurons also have their own switching mechanisms, which turn on and off the various functions of that particular organ.

One of the key harmonic expressions of these clock genes and SCN cells are the neurotransmitter-hormones melatonin and serotonin. The major on and off switches for these biochemicals include light along with a biochemical switching (inhibitory) neurotransmitter messenger called GABA (Gamma-aminobutyric acid) (Perreau-Lenz *et al.* 2005). The dense network of serotonergic neurons within the central nervous system connects with networks of SCN cells. Light-driven oscillations of the SCN cells thus stimulate rhythmic serotonin release through these neurons' activity (Moore and Speh 2004).

The photoreceptor signaling process is still somewhat mysterious, but it appears that a protein called malanopsin is involved in a photo pigmentation process stimulating SCN cells. The signaling transduction pathway proposed with respect to the gene phosphorylation system is Glu-Ca2+-CaMKII-nNOS-GC-cGMP-cGK – > – >clock genes. This is obviously a waveform transmission and semiconductance pathway. The body's crystalline transmission and reception sequences within DNA translate these waveforms into intelligent instructional signals.

In 2005, Dr. Erik Herzog and Sara Aton discovered a peptide that lies between SCN neurons, seemingly polarizing their rhythmic oscillations. The *vasoactive intestinal polypeptide* (VIP), so named because it was found in the gut, became noteworthy because it is apparently produced within the SCN cell pathway. Dr. Herzog proposed that the VIP lying between SCN neurons *"is like a rubber band between the pendulums of two grandfather clocks, helping to synchronize their timing"* (Aton *et al.* 2005).

Dr. Paolo Sassone-Corsi's 2006 studies at the University of California led to an understanding that CLOCK genes function quite like enzymes. A year later, Dr. Sassone-Corsi's research found that a single amino acid within the BAL1 protein provides the initial switching signal when it undergoes a single modification. That amino acid bonding modification stimulates the rest of the body clock's switching systems.

As researchers have delved deeper into the mystery of the body clock mechanisms, they have found increasingly complex signaling pathways, involving a myriad of biochemicals and gene sequences. The irony here is that scientists have been looking for a single biochemical or gene that is somehow ultimately responsible for the body's clock system. Instead, soon after one biochemical, molecule or gene is located and thought to be the clock mechanism; another seems to emerge. The apparent weakness seems to be in the theory of one particular clock mechanism. In reality, most of our body functions in a clockwork fashion, with every molecule, cell and tissue system processing to related rhythms.

One mystery illustrating the weakness of the single biochemical switch theory is that blind people have functional biological clocks. A blind body's clockworks will tune precisely to the sun's clockworks despite no obvious entry of light to the pineal gland's SCN region. It has been proposed that retinal cells contain another type of neural photoreceptor system – one receiving electromagnetic rhythms outside the visual relay system. Another theory proposes that a few photoreceptor cells remain in blind people. This allows the stimulation of the pineal/SCN system without enough impulses to stimulate the LGN and visual cortex.

A larger mystery is how these various clockwork genes and cells communicate and synchronize throughout the body. In 2004, Dr. David Welsh and a team of researchers observed individual fibro-blasts under various conditions. Fibroblasts are cells that will differentiate into connective tissue cells, osteoblasts and other cells. It turns out that fibroblasts also contain self-regulating circadian clockwork genes. They somehow synchronize their behavior with the rest of the rhythmic activities of the body.

Imagine a house full of thousands of clocks, each having differ-ent timing mechanisms and different alarms, dials, pacing, and functioning. Then imagine every one resetting automatically to the same time when signaled by one. With this, we might take a step toward understanding the fantastic array of synchronization neces-sary to coordinate all of the body's various clocks.

A good example is the cycle between cortisol and melatonin. Each is driven by different cascading pathways. Cortisol – known to increase metabolism – tends to increase and peak as melatonin – known to decrease metabolism and induce sleep – recedes in the early morning. Then, after a couple of daytime cycles, cortisol levels recede in the evening and melatonin levels increase correspondingly. Melatonin peaks around midnight as the cortisol levels have dropped completely. Here independent biochemical pathways are driven by seemingly independent endocrine systems. Somehow, these cycles synchronize with each other, yet do not overlap. Through some entrainment mechanism, one gradually recedes while the other increases. This single feat, repeated billions of times every second, is orchestrated. What is the orchestrating mechanism? What provides the baseline direction or controlling purpose?

The Solar Circadian Clock

Circadian rhythms cycle and recur daily, synchronized with the sun's relative path through our sky. The timing of the human body clock's solar day, however, will also vary to the various rhythmic cues of our immediate environment and physiology. As infants, we begin life in the body tied to the rhythms of our mother. As we emerge from the womb, our bodies begin their entrainment to the sun's path. This entrainment process takes a little time. Infants progress from almost all day sleep (with some feeding and crying in between) to sleep precisely timed to the sun. Gradually, the frequency of daytime sleep decreases. Not randomly, mind you. Rather, a baby's sleep cycles decrease in daily frequency at a consistent pattern, influenced by geographical location (with respect to the equator) and the amount of artificial light present in the room. In other words, with each passing sunrise and sunset, our bodies slowly and gradually entrain their rhythms to nature's cycles. By the time our bodies reach adolescence, our clocks have become quite rigid, exhaustively trained by so many daily cycles of the sun.

Over the past forty years, sleep researchers have been rigorously studying our entrained circadian clocks by incubating and isolating people, animals and cells. This has been accomplished variously, using caves and isolated chambers with and without the benefit of light. A host of mechanisms related to the body's circadian clockworks has been proposed. Various studies done with and without interaction with light have shown that melatonin rises with the dimming of lights. Melatonin levels also tend to fall with the body's interaction with even a little light. Core body temperature also appears to be a major component of the melatonin surge. As the body cools with the dimming of lights in the evening, melatonin begins to pulse into the bloodstream. In the early evening, cortisol levels peak and then begin to fall off with body core temperature, guiding the body into slumber. As cortisol begins its rise around 3am, body core temperature begins to increase, as our body gradually prepares itself for a new day of activity.

Our rhythmic anatomy is designed to revolve around the sun's path. The sun's path orchestrates the body's rhythms through the activity of the pineal gland, the SCN cells and various clockwork genes, which all resonate throughout the body. Receiving light through the eyes appears critical to the pineal's response. Yet light still seems to stimulate the pineal with the eyes closed or blinded. Most assuredly there are various other receptors around the body that respond to the sun's waveforms as well. Therefore, we can surmise that it is the electromagnetic activity of the sun – not merely the visible light spectrum – that lies at the heart of the sun's influence upon the body. The sun's electromagnetic waveform mechanisms also adjust the body's rhythms on a daily basis. These adjustments are expressed through physiological biochemical pathways, which stimulate the secretion and activity of the various hormones, neurotransmitters and their receptors.

Cave studies like Kleitman (1963), Foer and Siffre (2008), and Miles *et al.* (1977) have indicated the human body's daily revolution – without the resetting mechanism of daylight – is about 24.9 hours. This exact period has been debated, as researchers have also seen body rhythms cycle variously. These and other isolation studies conducted over weeks without daily light cues revealed that while temperature cycles may approach twenty-four hours long, sleep cycles can stretch out to as long as thirty hours. They indicated that over time, the body clock tends to deform without the sun. They also indicated that we each have unique responses to a lack of daily sun. Without the daily resetting mechanism of the sun, we might be going to bed later and later each night. After a few weeks, we might find ourselves doing all-nighters and sleeping during the daytime.

The consistent issue among these various studies on the body clock is how predictably the body's clockworks mechanisms reset with sunlight. For example, Dr. Czeisler performed studies (Kelly *et al.* 1989) with the Naval Health Research Center on Trident nuclear submarine crewmembers. Sub operation schedules required crew to attempt to maintain an 18-hour body clock. Dr. Czeisler's results found this just was not possible. The onboard lights were simply too weak to entrain their body clocks to that schedule. Dr. Czeisler and others have since established that bright light from between 7,000 and 13,000 (typical daylight) lux was necessary to produce a resetting of the body clock (Boivin *et al.* 1996).

The human body can also respond to lower intensities of light, however. In another study, Dr. Czeisler and Boivin (1998) studied eight healthy men with eight control subjects. They found a mere 180 lux of light (typical office lighting ranges from 200-400 lux) had the ability to shift the circadian body clock, together with an increase in body core temperature. In another test, Dr. Czeisler found that 100 lux of indoor light will have about half the alerting response as 9100 lux of outdoor light (Cajochen *et al.* 2000). In a study of twelve adults, Dr. Czeisler and his associates (Gronfier *et al.* 2007) found that while 100 lux is sufficient to shift the clock, a 25-lux light was not enough to shift or reset the body's clock.

We each have unique responses to light. In one study (Cajochen *et al.* 2003) done at Harvard's Brigham and Women's Hospital in 2003, 45% of the study population responded to 3.5 lux of light for 16 hours rotated with 0 lux during 8 hours of sleep. The rest responded to different lux levels. This report also concluded that the body's circadian clock appears to oscillate at between 23.9 and 24.5 hours – again negating the 25-hour body clock assumption.

We might present the opinion – held by many – that because most of the cave and isolation experiments required some indoor lighting for sanity's sake, many studies were unable to accurately measure the clock's subtle cuing tolerances. Dr. Czeisler and his associates have admitted that perhaps some of the body's rhythms are more rigid than others. For example, melatonin cycles appear to be more resistant to phase changes, although melatonin periods can vary when sleep schedules are adjusted (Boivin *et al.* 1996; Cajocken *et al.* 2003).

Sleep is irreparably tied to sunlight. After a couple of weeks in temporal isolation chambers – meaning with no sunlight, only artificial light and no time signals – subjects will sleep highly irregular hours. Some days a subject might sleep up to 19 hours a day, while other days the sleep length might be as few as four hours. Interestingly, on days with as little as four hours sleep, subjects did not recognize that they had too little sleep. They remained awake for as many as 30 hours in a row without apparent sleepiness (St Hilaire *et al.* 2007).

These studies have confirmed a circadian body clock exists, with a range from around 24 hours to 25 hours. However, this clock requires sunlight to stay on track. We do see a variance in the body clock time with the season of the study, the environment of the study, and study participants and protocols. Proximity to the equator, the phase of the moon, and the earth's rotation period all seem to have an effect as well. This indicates that the body's clockworks are subject to other influences besides the timing of sunrise and sunset – but the sun is still the main driving force.

The earth's rotation period also varies from 24 hours, and its clockwork is regulated by the sun's relative position. The earth's *sidereal* is approximately 23 hours, 56 minutes and 4.091 seconds. However when we consider the earth's rotation with respect to the sun, we arrive at closer to 24 hour cycles from setting sun to setting sun, adjusting for seasonal variance. Other cycles in nature are very similar in their slight variation from a static, atomic clock (this also varies, but infinitesimally). The rhythms of nature are moving through a myriad of cycles, creating incremental rhythms and interference patterns – all driven by the sun.

Slight variances in periods also provide just enough flexibility for choice. If all cycles were unchangeable and exact, we would be discussing machinery. Environmental variances allow for optional behavior, which allow the human organism to assess and select optional activities. Environmental variances and entrainment only affect entrainment to a certain degree. A person intending to stay up late to enjoy an evening with friends will force a governing factor onto the overall rhythm of their body's clock, for example.

There is also a cognition variable to consider in sunlight rhythms. Isolation chamber subjects will quickly become disoriented with respect to time once their light cues are taken away. Subjects may perceive that 2-3 weeks went by during a month, for example. Despite this confusion, subjects without sleep cues will typically make sleep adjustments in a cyclic way, eventually falling into a new rhythm. Even then, isolation-chamber subjects illustrate a residual 24-25 hour clock with variances cycling at a 127-day rhythm, whereupon their sleep rhythm cycles often return to a resetting rhythm driver.

The suprachiasmatic nuclei system helps entrain the body's rhythms to the waveforms of sunlight. SCN cells are a part of the pathway that regulates the timing and production of melatonin and cortisol. They also directly or indirectly influence thermo-regulation through thyroid hormones and various neurotransmitters. SCN cells, together with the clock genes, the pineal gland and hypothalamus, act as translation conveyers of sorts: Translating the slightly varying degrees of sunlight into the appropriate responses. The environmental components driven by the sun include visible light, heat, colors, light intensity and magnetism.

A number of hormones, such as thyroid hormones, estrogen and testosterone cycle with solar periodicity. Melatonin appears to be the principle solar rhythm hormone, however. As the pineal gland reacts to the absence of the sun's electromagnetic radiation, it stimulates the production of this pervading hormone.

The chemical synthesis of melatonin begins with a hydroxylation of tryptophan to 5-hydroxytryptophan, which decarboxylates to serotonin. Serotonin is then converted to N-acetylserotonin, which is methylated to melatonin. Melatonin affects the cellular biological clock and metabolism in a myriad of ways. Melatonin is involved in the signaling of puberty and related sex hormone levels; the stimulation of the immune system; the constriction of blood vessels; the modulation and release of various mood hormones like dopamine and serotonin; and numerous other metabolic functions.

Another biochemical related to sleep is adenosine. Like melatonin, adenosine levels rise in the bloodstream relative to the absence of the sun. With the alternation of sunlight with darkness, these two biochemicals alternate with cortisol, testosterone, epinephrine and thyroid hormones. Melatonin and adenosine are also part of the signalling pathways that promote cooling the body. Body core temperature is slowed as cellular metabolism slows. Lower body temperature also provides the basis for a neural feedback loop confirming that the body is ready for a sleep.

The artificial suns of today's modern electric world discourage the body's melatonin and adenosine release. Lights with even moderate lux levels have been shown to lower circulating melatonin levels. By design, our bodies produce less melatonin if the lights are left on too long after sunset, because lights signal to the body a need to keep working. Late night lighting increases circulating levels of cortisol. Over time, this can exhaust the adrenal glands – critical to the release of cortisol and other corticosteroids.

Deficient melatonin levels have been linked to lowered immunity and heightened rates of cancer and other diseases. A number of pro-inflammatory cytokines are produced when the body is not sleeping enough or is operating on an irregular cycle. Pro-inflammatory interleukin-6 is one of these, and its release correlates with irregular sleep patterns. Another pro-inflammatory trigger, tumor necrosis factor (TNF), is typically higher in persons with inadequate or irregular sleep cycles. Heightened levels of these cytokines have been particularly evident during daytime sleepiness episodes (Vgontzas *et al.* 2005).

About 90% of our body's melatonin production is eventually metabolized out of the body through the liver. Since there are a number of other hormones related to core body temperature that revolve around the body's circadian rhythms – including thyroid hormones, growth hormones, adrenaline and others – it is safe to conclude that melatonin is not the driver of the body's sleeping clockworks. Rather, the sun is the ultimate driver.

Indeed, many other hormones and metabolic cycles rotate in synchronicity with circadian rhythms. All are also directly or indirectly entrained to the sun.

For example, men have a number of distinct circadian hormone cycles. Few realize just how important hormone regulation is to men's moods and physical status. Research on males over the past decade has confirmed circadian patterns among testosterone, aldosterone, luteinizing hormone and inhibin B. A Russian study by Pronina (1992) on males in five different age groups determined that all of these hormones cycled through the day. Rhythm amplitudes of aldosterone and testosterone peaked highest in seven to eight year old boys, while LH rhythm amplitudes peaked highest among thirteen and fourteen year old adolescent boys.

In another study (Carlsen *et al.* 1999), thirteen healthy males were tested every 30 minutes for inhibin B – a glycoprotein thought to be a feedback-inhibiting messenger for FSH secretion. Significant daily cycles were noted, with peak values of inhibin B in the morning, and lower values in the afternoon and evening. Inhibin B levels cycled opposite those of testosterone and estradiol.

Morning testosterone levels appear to be associated positively with the amount of sleep a male gets the night before (Penev 2007). Other hormones – such as growth hormone – have shown to be related not only to sleep quantity, but also to sleep quality.

In a study of 149 men aged between 16 and 83 years old, growth hormone levels and cortisol levels were studied concurrent with brainwave sleep analysis. Regardless of age, daily growth hormone levels slowed as the amount of slow brainwave sleep decreased. The less slow wave sleep the person had, the lower the amount of growth hormone the person produced. This trend also occurred in an age-related basis: The older the man, the less slow brainwave sleep he had, and thus the lower growth hormone production (Van Cauter *et al.* 2000).

Slow brainwave sleep is of course related to heightened levels of melatonin, relaxation, and enough sleep time. These all tie to sleeping with the sun's rhythms, as melatonin is related to darkness.

The relationship between daily cortisol levels in the Van Cauter study also related to sleep quality. Rapid eye movement sleep or REM sleep was associated negatively with evening cortisol levels among the subjects. In other words, independent of age, less REM sleep equated to more evening cortisol. However, this trend also did occur with age: The older men had progressively lower REM sleep and thus higher evening cortisol levels. This in turn would also reduce melatonin levels, thereby keeping core body temperatures up and lowering sleep quality. Both higher cortisol levels and lower REM sleep are directly related to stress. This is consistent with other sleep studies confirming that adults get less REM sleep as we age – likely relating to stress and dysfunctional rhythms.

In one study (Evans *et al.* 2007), fifty active seniors at the University of Westminster were continuously measured for cortisol levels through a forty-eight hour period in their homes. Before and after exams showed that ultradian cortisol cycles significantly correlated with changing impressions of psychological well-being. This was significant during the first 45 minutes after awaking from sleep. Those with lower morning cortisol tended to experience increased feelings of well-being, for example.

Many other daily secretions are not only circadian, but are affected by stressors such as reduced sleep and increased occupational stress. In one study (Persson *et al.* 2006) of 75 workers, those who involuntarily worked over 80 hours in a week experienced dysfunctional levels of cholesterol, cortisol, melatonin, prolactin, and testosterone levels on day seven of the workweek. In fact, both groups (the 40-hour workers and the 80-plus-hour workers) experienced decreased levels at the end of the workweek when compared to the beginning of the workweek. This would suggest that these hormones and neurotransmitters decrease with more stress and reduced outdoor activity. This would be consistent with research illustrating that reduced or low-quality sleep is linked with a reduction in sunlight exposure. The stimulation of hormones and neurotransmitters that balance and alternate with sleep hormones like adenosine and melatonin require healthy sunlight exposure.

Ultradian Cycling

The sun's daily cycle drives a multitude of cycles throughout the day. Ultradian cycles have periods of less than a day. Circadian rhythms cross over and influence most ultradian rhythms. These intersections influence just about every metabolic function within the body. These include cellular metabolism, respiration, cardiovascular function, digestion, thirst, body core temperature regulation, moods, cognition and many others.

Ultradian cycles vary to the organism. Metabolic cycles among yeasts range from thirty to ninety minutes long, while transcriptional cell division processes cycle at about forty minutes (Lloyd and Murray 2007). Complex organisms display an even greater number of ultradian cycles each day. Ultradian neurotransmitter cycles in humans are connected not only with changes in metabolism and thermoregulation, but also with our changing moods and habits throughout the day. Some hormone and neurotransmitter cycles are circadian, and some cycle in smaller ultradian rhythms.

For most of us, by around three a.m. our adrenal cortex begins to quietly pump cortisol into the bloodstream. With cortisol comes higher body core temperatures and increased metabolism amongst the cells. This process subtly orchestrates our multiple sleep cycles – which are also ultradian. Our body slowly comes out of its low-activity deep sleep state, gliding into a lighter cycle in anticipation of awaking. Cortisol levels gradually build close to dawn. They tend to peak a few hours after daybreak.

Should the sunrise not be synchronized with our first cortisol cycle, we will find our last few hours sleep is less restful. Getting quality sleep after dawn is increasingly difficult by design, because sunlight stimulates increased levels of cortisol, adrenaline and testosterone.

After waking in the morning, these levels should increase as our body temperature rises. Our cortisol surge should peak about an hour or two after waking, tapering off towards the late morning, accompanied by a late-morning decline in energy. This cycle of lower energy continues into the early afternoon as our bodies head into 'siesta' mode (researchers call this the *lunch challenge*). After a digestive cycle-down, cortisol levels again tend to rise. Depending upon our exposure to the sun, eating habits, stressors, and environment; another rise in cortisol – not usually as high as the morning's – will begin sometime in the middle to late afternoon.

Cortisol levels will also rise during times of stress or urgency. This spike can occur at any time of day, and it will usually be accompanied by increases in other stress biochemicals. These include norepinephrine, acetylcholine, and others, which help orchestrate changes in metabolism to respond to the urgency. These will facilitate increased blood flow and nutrients to the muscles, eyes and brain cells, with a decrease in blood flow and nutrients to organs like the liver, immune system and the digestive system. They will also facilitate other neurotransmitters such as epinephrine. For this reason, a physiology pushed by constant stress will usually result in digestive issues, liver problems and lowered immunity.

An abundance of these stressful or anxious responses over extended periods (called *chronic stress*) combined with reduced sun exposure will result in lower morning cortisol levels. This will usually lower energy throughout the day. This condition is often diagnosed as *chronic fatigue syndrome* or *fibromyalgia*, often traced to underproductive adrenal glands.

Given continuous light exposure, later afternoon and early evening cortisol levels again rise. This gives us a burst of energy at the end of the day and into the early evening. The extent of ultradian cortisol secretion and the amplitude (or slope) of the cortisol cycle is related to internal and external environmental conditions in addition to conscious factors. These include levels of estrogen, lutein phase, inflammation, physical fitness, weather, sound, color, oxygen, anxiety and of course, sunlight exposure.

A number of other ultradian cycles are working in conjunction with the sun: Most also interact (or interfere) with our metabolic cycles. For example, multiple daily temperature fluctuations were illustrated among babies by Bollani *et al.* (1997). In a study on cognition by Klein and Armitage (1979), it was shown that study participants' verbal and spatial skills cycled at about ninety-six minutes. Other studies have confirmed several other body rhythms that rotate at intervals close to 90 minutes each. The length of these rhythms correlate closely with the close-to-ninety minute cycles of REM and non-REM stage sleeping pattern, as documented over many years of government-sponsored sleep research led by William Dement, M.D. (1999).

Research has connected brainwaves with the various ultradian rhythms occurring throughout the body. Brainwaves are also ultradian. Slower brainwave rhythms have been connected with the neural activity within the thalamus and cerebral cortex. An oscillation of *spindle complexes* among these ganglia pathways drive rhythmic pulses through the brain, reverberating throughout the body (Burikov and Bereshpolova 1999). These complex switching neurons have been called *corticothalamic* neurons, and they transduce slow delta waves (Timofeev and Steriade 1996).

Meanwhile, the faster alpha waves reverberating through our bodies are connected to the optic nerve response of visual input through the LGN to the visual cortex. This function has been tested by reading subjects' brainwave responses in the occipital region while they were visual recognizing particular shapes and sizes. With the processing of visual information, alpha waves were generated (Shevelev *et al.* 1991). Alpha waves may thus be regarded as indicative of imagery and sunlight reflected on the visual cortex' scanning process.

The slower theta rhythms, moving at between four and ten cycles per second, are associated with relaxation, sleep and sunlight exposure. In waking adults, theta waves are crowded out by focused consciousness. Some tests have shown that theta waves will still occur with certain short-term memory tasks; episodic and semantic memory recalls; and spatial navigation tasks (Buzsaki 2005). Relaxation and semantic memory recall require thoughts of a more abstract basis. These slower waveforms are thus reflective of deeper, more abstract awareness. Several studies of theta waves have concluded that they appear to reflect activity related to the functions of the hippocampus – a central player in the human limbic system. Theta waves have also been linked with rhythmic movement like dancing, along with certain auditory processing during both waking and sleeping. They have also been observed during attention shifting (Gambini *et al.* 2002).

The somewhat mysterious theta rhythm may also provide a link to the programming mechanisms required for autonomic function. Pedemonte and Velluti (2005) found that theta rhythms substantially affect the heart rate and many reflex movements, including programmed functions related to responsive memory. Theta waves are more pronounced around sunset and sunrise.

Hunger and appetite are ultradian rhythms to consider in the mix. These appear to be intimately connected to the workings of the hypothalamus. The hypothalamus is considered one of the centers for pleasure feedback among the limbic system components. The hypothalamus is activated by sensual interactions that include the feedback of taste, the olfactory sense, and the entrainment of eating cycles with sunlight exposure.

These together drive the flow of gastric juices. Sensual impulses from our olfactory nerves and organoleptic taste buds stimulate the vagus nerve. This in turn accelerates peristalsis and the production of acids from the stomach's gastric cells, along with amylase from our salivary glands. The secretion of bile from our gallbladder into our upper intestines follows shortly thereafter.

Over the past few decades, the study of America's two prime epidemics – obesity and diabetes – has driven researchers to better understand the biochemical messengers involved in the hunger/appetite/satiation cycle. This has unveiled a number of biochemical feedback-response mechanisms bridging solar rhythms with the limbic system, the stomach, the pancreas, fat cells and working cells.

The organs have their own ultradian rhythms. For example, Nobel Prize winner Dr. Alexis Carrel proposed in 1912 that rather than the heart being a pump – as it was thought of for the previous millennia – it is more like a turbine, working conjunctively with blood flow and artery pressure. Dr. Carrel's groundbreaking research on the heart is what ushered medicine into the era of open-heart surgery many years later. The rhythmic ebb and flow of the body's fluids – its blood, lymph, urine, digestive juices and others – appear unrelated when we focus on any one. Observed together, however, their relative cycles illustrate an orchestration between metabolism and the rhythms of the solar system.

Insulin, for example – a hormone produced by the beta cells of the pancreas – stimulates cells to become glucose-sensitive, stimulating their utilization of glucose from the bloodstream. Without a natural supply of this valuable hormone, the cells are starved for glucose, even if the bloodstream and liver is saturated with glucose and derivatives. This in turn opens the door to various cardiovascular, circulatory, cognitive and liver-related health problems. Western society's epidemic of adult-onset diabetes – no longer "adult-onset" – relates to insulin and glucose receptor sensitivity at the cell membrane. Insulin production, it turns out, is only a small part of the biochemical signalling mechanisms using a host of ligands and receptors.

Insulin production is related to a number of other signalling biochemicals that manage energy consumption. These include leptin, ghrelin, resistin, adiponectin, cholecystokinins, sirtuins and others. These cycle with the energy needs of the body, which in turn cycle with sleep, work, and other activities relating to the timing of sun exposure.

The hormone cascade is triggered from the pineal gland's responses to the light of the sun. The pineal gland in turn triggers a response in the hypothalamus. The hypothalamus releases neurotransmitters that stimulate the anterior pituitary with timed releasing hormones. These releasing hormones stimulate the pituitary to release master hormones that drive the endocrine system. For example, ACTH hormones stimulate the adrenal gland to release glucocorticoids. The pituitary's release of TSH hormone stimulates the thyroid to produce secondary hormones T3 and T4, which help maintain metabolic balance.

This hormonal relay process is more than just automatic. It is informational. For example, certain pituitary hormone messages will suppress T3 release while elevating rT3 levels during physical stress. Other hormone messengers will reverse this process. These types of interactive signals are coordinated through switching and feedback mechanisms – which relay information from internal and external conditions. As the body's physical and environmental conditions change, some hormone releases are shunted by other signal-ling mechanisms (Mastorakos and Pavlatou 2005).

The relationship between thyroid hormone and the cell's utiliza-tion of glucose with insulin becomes evident in the case of hyperthyroidism. Most hyperthyroidism cases also present with increased metabolic activity, causing an increase in the conversion of glucose into energy and lactate (Dimitriadis and Raptis 2001). This illustrates how easily the interruption or over stimulation of the normal thyroid cycle and T3 production can cause a negative domino effect – increasing glucose and insulin needs, appetite, binge eating, and weight gain.

Thyroid hormone is directly related to sun exposure. Thyroid signalling is intimately related to the flow of melatonin. Melatonin levels are regulated through a handshaking between the hypothala-mus and pineal gland as they respond to light reduction – as we've discussed. Along with this cyclic melatonin release, thyroid hor-mones T3 and T4 cycle in shifts cooperating with the corticoster-oids – all entrained to the passage of the sun (Wright 2002).

The rhythms of the sun also intertwine with other ultradian cy-cles. Consider the beating of the heart and the pacing of respiration. Most of us have experienced how an increase in heat or physical activity will increase the heart rate and the rate of breathing simultaneously. These are managed by a set of synchronized bio-chemicals that include vasopressin and angiotensin. These relate to the pressure differentials between water content, oxygen and carbon dioxide levels, stress, heart rate and other considerations. They also relate to the arterial walls' ability to respond to changing environ-mental conditions with expansion or contraction (vasodilation and vasoconstriction). They also directly relate to the functions of the kidneys, the liver, the heart, the blood vessels and endocrine system. They also interact with the conversion of glucose, oxygen and min-erals to energy within mitochondria; in a complex process called the *Krebs cycle*. Vasopressin is released by the pituitary gland, which is stimulated by the pineal gland, which is stimulated by sunlight.

These are all intertwined with body core temperature fluctua-tions and the reception of light by the pineal gland. The thermal dynamics of the body cycle in a regulatory process called *homeostasis*. Homeostasis is the process the body undergoes to keep its temperature balanced. Should body core temperature rise or fall below the range of about 95 degrees F to 104 F, the body's metabolic balance will be challenged. If it is too cold, various enzymatic functions will slow. If it is too hot, the cells can become overheated, causing exhaustion and muscle fatigue. Thermoregulation is a balancing act, keeping the various interactive processes tuned to a particular thermal range. In a healthy body, temperature rhythms synchronize to slightly rise and fall throughout the day with the rise and fall of cortisol and melatonin. These rhythms form a pervasive biofeedback-response loop, together with thyroid hormones to result in a relatively balanced body core temperature range whether it is hot or cold in the outside environment. This mechanism connects metabolic temperature to the electromagnetic and thermal output of the sun and relative seasonal position of the sun in the sky.

Should we plot temperature, metabolism and levels of most of these biochemical mechanisms over a day's time, we would find most cycle in a manner similar to the shape of a sine wave. Furthermore, as the various environmental and physiological cycles are examined together, we find they interact coherently. During coherence, cycles with constructive interference provide mechanisms for ion channel gate opening, while destructive interference provides mechanisms for ion channel gate closing. Just as the magnetic portion of the electromagnetic wave pushes outward and perpendicular from the plane of the electronic vector, these interlocked body cycles all effect the biological environment of the body in an alternating vector, expanding heat and motion cycles ancillary to the functional metabolic cycles.

An interesting example of this multi-dimensional field of coherence is the peristalsis cycle of the gastrointestinal system. Peristalsis is a series of rhythmic contractions of the smooth muscles that govern the size and shape of the digestive tract. This tract includes the esophagus, the stomach, the small intestine, the colon and the anus, along with supporting muscle groups and organs. If we were to examine the frequency of peristaltic contraction of smooth muscle around each intestinal region, we would find that each paces with a different rhythm. Because the process of digestion within each component has a different mechanism, the frequency of the cycles within each component is different. Around the stomach, peristaltic waves occur from three to eight times per minute (or 180 to 480 cycles per second). Throughout the intestine, peristaltic waves vibrate at a rhythm of ten to twenty times per minute (600 to 1200 hertz). In the colon, peristaltic waves move in the same range as the stomach – from 180 to 480 hertz – yet will typically maintain a different wavelength and amplitude from that of the stomach.

Peristaltic waves are considered "slow waves." These waves are driven by fluctuations in electronic potential. Smooth muscle resting potential ranges from -50 to -60 mV. A partial depolarization of these muscle fibers causes a fluctuation of membrane potential of 5 to 15 mV. This electronic fluctuation of potential causes muscle contraction when the potential spikes.

Peristaltic waves escort food through the esophagus, massaging its entry into the cavity of the stomach and intestines. There are two primary functions involved here: The propulsion of the food, and the mixing of food with enzymes and gastrin. The first wave that massages food from the esophagus to the stomach typically lasts from 8-9 seconds. Secondary waves will continue as the bolus (partially digested food and digestive juices) mixes in the stomach, accompanied by peristaltic waves of faster frequencies. These faster peristaltic waves liquefy the food mixing in the stomach.

Guiding the propulsion and mixing process are two interneuron reflex systems that release neurotransmitters into the neurons that stimulate the smooth muscles. The first is a group of excitatory motor neurons stimulated above the bolus. These nerves initiate the contraction of the smooth muscles using neurotransmitters acetylcholine and substance P as messengers. The second nerve group is inhibitory. These nerves stimulate the relaxation of the muscles below the bolus, allowing the bolus to pass through. This second group of neurons is driven by released neurotransmitters such as vasoactive intestinal peptide and nitric oxide.

As the bolus (now together with chyme) moves through the pyloric valve and into the intestines, peristaltic waves continue to provide the motion to encourage the bolus downward as nutrients are being absorbed through the intestinal wall. Eventually, the insoluble fiber and chyme will be moved into the colon, where it is mixed with other biochemicals and liver byproducts, and dehydrated and prepared for evacuation. Both longitudinal and circular muscle fibers are engaged alternatively around the intestines and colon. Much of this takes place through a process of local longitudinal shortening, which shortens the longitudinal muscles, and increases circular muscle tone.

As the bolus stretches each portion of the digestive tract, neurotransmitters are released into the smooth muscle. This sensitizes the muscle with the greater membrane potential. As the cyclic peristaltic wave passes over that area, the muscle fibers contract, followed by relaxation. This alternating contraction and relaxation process cumulatively moves food through the digestive tract, and provides a precision of mixing among bile, probiotics and enzymes. The viability of our probiotic systems – essential to health, depends upon peristaltic wave coherence.

The relationships between sunshine and the rhythmic activities of the digestive tract illustrate how the body's cycles are intertwined with nature's cycles. As is with any harmonic relationship, affecting one aspect will have a reflective effect on those other cyclic activities functioning in conjunction.

The interruption of any one of the body's rhythms by the removal of regular sunlight exposure, or the introduction of synthetic hormones, gastric inhibitors, neurotransmitter receptor agonists or antagonists – or practically any other type of interference with the body's rhythmic flow of hormones, metabolism, reproduction, digestion, and so on – will create an imbalance elsewhere to be reconciled. The imbalanced unnatural lifestyle of the modern world creates the unfortunate consequence of having to deal with increasingly new disorders and consequences that we had previously not even imagined let alone predicted. The onslaught of various new pathologies over the past few decades including new allergies, fibromyalgia, food sensitivities, autoimmune disorders and various cancers are all signs that our body's rhythmic coherences are being stressed. This is not to say a lack of sunlight is the only form of attack on our various rhythmic mechanisms. Within today's environment are so many synthetic toxins, ranging from plasticizers to toxicity in our air and water.

An important aspect of our body's rhythmic mechanisms is the element of uniqueness. Every body is tuned to relatively the same major external stimuli. Yet every body is unique. Each cycles slightly differently to the same external stimuli. One body might thus respond quickly and intensely to a particular stressor. Another body might resist such a response, maintaining its cycles with hardly any alteration. While genes certainly play a role, this ultimately stems from each body containing an individual personality.

Still, we find many metabolic cycles common among healthy people. Feeling hungry and eating multiple times per day, sleeping six to eight hours per night and so on. Adaptogenic mechanisms uniquely smooth out any incongruities. For example, should we feel fatigued due to overexertion, a good night's sleep will stimulate our body's various repair systems to heal the damage. Should we wake up with the sun the next day, our metabolic processes and hormonal rhythms will likely be readjusted and refreshed. One body might require 7.25 hours to achieve this readjustment. Another might require 8 hours. Still another might require 9 hours to regain strength, and still more the next night.

Many of us consider that our body clocks are permanent. Subsequently we figure we are either "evening people" or "morning people" for the body's duration, for example. What we may not realize is that the conscious choices we make involving our activities and dietary choices greatly influence our body rhythms. The subsequent production of cortisol, melatonin, thyroid hormones, sex hormones, growth hormones and the other daily cyclic biochemical flows all tune into and respond individually to an environment timed to the sun's rhythms.

The relationships between our decisions and our body cycles were illustrated in a study of 1,572 children from fourth to eighth grades (Gau *et al.* 2004). Children who reported they were "evening people" were more likely to drink coffee and have less parental monitoring. These "evening people" children stayed up later, and experienced increased moodiness and daytime sleepiness (and most certainly reduced sunlight exposure). It is probably fair to say that once we disturb our natural body rhythms entrained by the sun's path, we find that our moods, energy levels and metabolic body cycles (including sleep) become deranged.

The 5,000-year-old science of *Ayurveda* – translated as "the science of life" – recognized these daily ultradian rhythms. In

Ayurveda, the day is broken up into six three-hour ultradian cycles; each predominated by an alternating of one of the three *dosha* behaviors, *kapha, pitta* or *vata.* The three hours before 11pm, and three hours during mid-morning are each considered dominated by the *kapha* aspect in *Ayurveda.* The mid-day through the afternoon, and the three hours late after about 11 pm through about 2 am are considered governed by the *pitta* aspect. Just before and just after dawn and dusk are considered *vata* periods.

During each of these daily periods, certain activities are said to naturally prevail. Particular foods and liquids are suggested during each period as well. For example, spiced tea, water, and non-mucus-forming foods are said to be good for the morning *kapha* period, while fasting is suggested for the nighttime *kapha* (when we should be sleeping). The heaviest meal of the day is suggested during the *pitta* noon period – when digestive fires are thought to be at their peak. Meanwhile, grain-based meals are suggested for the post-sunset *vata* period and the after-sunrise *vata* period. The pre-sunrise and pre-sunset *vata* periods are also considered significant times for reflection, meditation and prayer in *Ayurveda.* Exercise is recommended by *Ayurveda* during the *pitta* and *kapha* periods of the day, depending upon the type of exercise.

Within these six governing periods, the Ayurvedic science divides the circadian day and night into thirty *ghatikas,* replacing the more arbitrary twelve-hour clock. Each *ghatika* is twenty-four minutes long. In the *ghatika* system, every day and every night consists of six sections of five *ghatikas* each. These appear to uniquely intersect the rhythms of nature's elements and those of the human body. The twenty-four minute rhythm also ties in very well with the estimated forty-five and ninety-minute sleep and REM cycles. Two cycles of 24 minutes equates roughly with the 45-minute and 90-minute sleep cycles, rounded to plus-or-minus five to ten minutes. Coincidence?

These are just a few of the body rhythms and inter-relationships between nature's rhythms laid out in *Ayurveda.* We find many other cycles documented by this elegant and ancient human science – incidentally also considered one of the safest medical systems in practice today.

Infradian Rhythms

The rhythms of the body that cycle over days, weeks and months have been the subject of study and controversy for thousands of years. Various Greek, Egyptian, Chinese and Ayurvedic physicians all saw the clockworks of the universe harmonizing with multiple daily and seasonal rhythms of the body. Hippocrates addressed this topic in his teachings, suggesting that physicians remain attentive to the good and bad days of their patients. Other famous early physicians such as Galen also recognized rhythms in health.

Western science began to take notice of infradian rhythms when Dr. Hermann Swoboda, a psychologist and professor at the University of Vienna in the early part of the twentieth century – investigated observations of periodic appearances of fevers, swelling, cardiac events, and other illnesses among his patients. Dr. Swoboda's painstaking recordkeeping methodology uncovered a 23-day physical cycle and a 28-day emotional cycle among his patients. Dr. Swoboda recorded his experiments and results in a number of German books on the subject: *The Periodicity in Man's Life; Studies on the Basis of Psychology; The Critical Days of Man;* and *The Year of Seven,* in which Dr. Swoboda elaborated on the mathematical and clinical foundation of these two cycles.

Dr. Wilhelm Fliess – another late nineteenth and early twentieth century physician most known for his work with Sigmund Freud – was the president of the German Academy of Sciences in 1910. Dr. Fliess began to study daily body cycles amongst his patients as well. Through detailed recordings and mathematical record keeping, Dr. Fliess independently came up with an identical theory: The body cycled through 23-day physical and 28-day emotional cycles. Dr. Fliess was a prolific writer, and recorded his studies in several scientific papers and gave numerous lectures. His books included the translated-from-German titles, *The Year in the Living, The Theory of Periodicity,* and *The Course of Life.*

Due to the elaborate research of Fliess and Swoboda, the controversial modern theory of *biorhythms* was born. Both Fliess and Swoboda unveiled an impressive array of statistics: Hundreds of family tree histories, numerous case studies; sibling studies; medical treatments; psychological events; traumas; accidents; and historical events were meticulously analyzed to establish these two cycles. The theories were controversial and many researchers of the day were skeptical. Still, many physicians and psychiatrists utilized the two cycles in their daily practice.

In the 1920s, mathematician and engineer Dr. Alfred Teltseher began to observe another pattern among his high school students. Dr. Teltseher launched an extensive analysis of what he called an *intellectual cycle*. His research revealed an apparent 33-day cycle of intellectual performance peaks, valleys, and critical days. Periods where learning is accelerated or delayed, periods of memory recall, and other periodic mental criteria were statistically examined by Dr. Teltseher among student performance and examinations. His scientific paper on the subject also correlated periodic endocrine secretions alongside Dr. Teltseher's 33-day intellectual cycle period (West 1999).

A decade later, Dr. Rexford Hersey and Dr. Michael Bennett reported a 35-36 day cycle of intellectual performance by studying railroad workers. The paper was picked up by Colgate University's Donald Laird, who reviewed the research in a paper titled *The Secrets of Our Ups and Downs,* which appeared in a science journal along with *Readers Digest* in August of 1935. Dr. Hersey spent many years thereafter studying this cycle, which included measuring the life statistics of nearly 5,000 men from 1927 to 1954 – providing the data for his 36-day cycle hypothesis (Crawley 1996).

These apparent cycles have been accumulated and elucidated by a number of writers over the past few decades. Each biocycle is described as a classic sine wave with a beginning point at the zero baseline and a high phase peak one-quarter through the cycle. This follows with a crossing of the zero baseline halfway through the cycle, a negative peak three-quarters through, and ending at the starting point of the zero baseline. Interestingly, the focus is not upon the high points and the low points of the cycle. Rather, the focus is upon the transition points, when the cycles cross the baseline, downward or upward. These transition points are termed *critical days*. The research mentioned above has indicated that these transition days – between the negative and the positive peaks on the curve – are apparently days when accidents or problems are more likely to occur.

In 1939, Swiss Federal Institute of Technology's Dr. Hans Schwing published a 78-page study of accidents and accidental deaths. This documented a pattern predicted by the three daily bio-wave cycles. His report consisted of a statistical analysis of 700 accident cases and 300 cases of accidental death. Dr. Schwing studied a period of 21,252 days, isolating critical days for the 23-day physical cycle, the 28-day emotional cycle, and the 33-day intellectual cycle. His report concluded that 322 accidents occurred during single critical days (in other words, one of the person's biorhythms were crossing the baseline into positive or negative territory); 72 occurred on double critical days (when two biorhythms are crossing the baseline); and five on triple critical days (when three biorhythms are crossing the baseline). A total of 401 accidents coincided with critical days, or 60% of all the accidents. The total number of critical days possible during the 21,252-day period was 4,427 days, or 20% of the 21,252 days. In other words, 60% of the accidents occurred on 20% of the possible days – those days coinciding with critical days.

A 1954 report by Rheinhold Bochow of Humboldt University in Berlin studied agricultural machinery accidents together with biorhythms. He found that out of 497 accidents, 97.8% of these took place on a critical day of one of the three body rhythms. Interestingly, 26.6% occurred on single critical days, 46.5% occurred on double critical days and 24.7% occurred on triple critical days. This seems to indicate that double critical days – an obviously rarer occasion than a single critical day in any biorhythm – are more dangerous than either single or triple critical days.

The link between these biorhythms and accidents has not been without its critics. Winstead *et al.* (1981) reported an analysis of potential biorhythm cycles with dates of psychiatric hospitalization and emergency room visits. They analyzed hospitalization dates for 218 patients and emergency room visits for 386 patients. No apparent correlations existed between these patients' biorhythms and critical biorhythm days. The authors of this study concluded the biorhythm theory is *"much too simplistic to account for the complexities of everyday life."*

Nonetheless, there is significant evidence to show human behavior and performance follows rhythmic patterns. Apparently, a number of companies in the transportation industry have reduced accident ratios using biorhythm critical day analysis in their risk assessments.

The negative phase of all three rhythms is known as a period of recovery and response rather than a period where lower performance or problems occur. As in all response periods, they also contribute to performance, however differently. For example, the response period for a cycle of breathing occurs when we breathe out. Some might consider this a negative flow relative to the input of oxygen during inspiration. This outflow is a necessary part of the cycle nonetheless – just as necessary as breathing in. Without expiration, carbon dioxide and carbolic acid levels would dangerously build up within the body. Rather, the theory of biorhythm performance says that the crossing from the negative or positive part of the cycle to the other – the critical day – in the midst of a breath – considered more critical.

The existence of biorhythm cycles is supported by recent research. According to biorhythm theory, the physical cycle in the positive phase should accompany a heightened sense of coordination and physical performance, along with faster recovery times. This has statistically been confirmed in many case studies of extraordinary performances among athletes. During this phase, the immune system should also be stronger, and thus disease resistance may be greater. Baran and Apostol (2007) studied various physical performance evaluations, revealing biorhythm intervals for tests such as neuromuscular efficiency.

While the Winstead research investigated psychiatric admissions, many diseases have illustrated distinct periodicity. For example, Leroux and Ducross (2008) reported that chronic cluster headaches have *"circannual and circadian periodicity."* A number of reports have linked various pathologies with different rhythms – many circadian and/or infradian. Respiration and airway resistance in asthma appears to have a rhythmic connection (Stephenson 2007). Incidence of breast cancer is linked with the body's rhythmic behavior (Sahar and Sassone-Corsi 2007). Chronic fatigue syndrome and its associated pain have been linked to infradian rhythms (Perrin 2007). Cardiac arrhythmias, ischemic heart disease and hypertension have all been linked to infradian rhythms (Portaluppi and Hermida 2007).

Arthritis has been linked to infradian cycles, particularly with respect to pro-inflammatory cytokines (Cutolo and Straub 2008).

Research also supports that communication, sensitivity and awareness may be better during the positive phase of the emotional cycle. Indeed, mood disorders have been positively linked with the body's rhythms in a number of studies (McClung 2007). Negotiations, exams, meetings, and team efforts may bring better results during a positive mental phase. The positive phase of an intellectual cycle also appears to bring stronger decision-making abilities. Learning ability has been shown to be heightened periodically. Studies on memory, executive function and attention capacity have also linked performance to infradian rhythms (Schmidt *et al.* 2007).

We should add that the rhythmic behaviors found in some of the above research were not necessarily reflecting the specific 23-day, 28-day, and 33-day biorhythm cycles. This growing database of research illustrates that so many metabolic activities are rhythmic, and these rhythms are all undoubtedly intertwined within the body and with the environmental rhythms brought on by the sun's activities. The confluence of these natural rhythms create significant interference patterns and intersecting points of metabolic activity. They are worth serious consideration in medicine.

Most researchers might agree that the body's systems fluctuate on rhythmic cycles. Pinpointing a strictly common cycle for everyone has proved problematic, however.

Assuming everyone precisely cycles to the same biorhythms, there is a rather easy calculation to make. To calculate our theoretical cycles to current, we would simply count the number of days since we were born, with a day added every leap year. We would then divide the total days of our lives by the number of days of each biorhythm. The remainder will be the number of days into the current biorhythm cycle. Again, this assumes we all cycle to precisely the same solar days.

It would appear likely that biorhythm cycles beginning on the day of birth would be subject to variances among the population just as so many other physical cycles are. The potential for cyclic variances seem likely given the proliferation of pre-term births, C-sections, delayed deliveries and other birth anomalies. In addition, we would suggest there is a significant range of events having the ability to influence our cycles. There could be so many possible variables. Logically we could apply one variance due to the location and time of day for our birth – whether this event took place at night under hospital lights, during the day out of doors or perhaps under the duress of an ambulance or even a rough car ride to the hospital. The trauma of a C-section or otherwise pre-term birth would likely apply particular stressors not normally existing in a natural birth as well. Certainly, a pre-term situation would affect the completion of the typical nine-month rhythm occurring for the fetus (incidentally an obvious infradian cycle for both the fetus and the mother). To this we would add the trauma of the birthing itself. Might these stressors affect the initiation or entrainment to a particular rhythm, just as the lack of sleep affects a person's daily entrainment to the sunrise?

The concurrence of various rhythmic occurrences – whether they are stress related, light related, or perhaps related to a particular trauma – should be considered as we analyze the variances among the critical day patterns. Dr. Schwing's 60% result for accident rates (out of a probability of 20%) may appeal to us scientifically. However, a 40% variance is also quite large when proposing we all cycle to the exact three same infradian rhythms. In other words, why did *all* of the accidents not occur on critical days? It appears unlikely that all of us each adhere to precisely the same rhythmic cycles, precisely beginning on the same day of our birth. We might add that humans could have cycled in closer proximity in the past than they might today, due to the prominence of natural childbirth and the adherence to natural sunlight as existed prior to a century ago. We extrapolate this because we know from circadian rhythm analysis that the sun's entrainment can significantly manage our circadian rhythms.

Rather, should we correlate solar entrainment with the many other known rhythmic disorders of the physical body (diabetes, obesity, insomnia, inflammation, and so on); we find a solid basis for concordance between disease and sun exposure – as we will discuss in detail later. We might consider the heart's rhythms, for example. If a person remains healthy with a good diet and a healthy amount of exercise, the heart rate should remain at a steady resting rate of 60-65 beats per minute during adulthood and possibly until advanced age. It would not be difficult to calculate this to beats-per-day and beats-per-year, establishing a solid pattern of rhythmicity quite similar to the calculation of the biorhythm cycles detailed earlier.

However, should we consider the rhythmicity of the heart in the case of an unhealthy diet, a chronic lack of exercise or a profuse amount of environmental stress, there is a likelihood the heartbeat rhythm could range from 65 to even 80 resting beats per minute. Obviously, the stressors applied to the physical body in the latter case changed both the rhythmicity and even the potential duration of the heart's lifetime. Some of this effect may well be outside of our control as well – should we find ourselves in a stressful occupation that required long hours and little sunlight, for example.

We see similar relationships between sun exposure and our body's natural rhythms. These include brainwaves, lifespan, sleep cycles, menstruation, and the many other rhythms that we have discussed so far.

There is no reason to believe the theoretical yet plausible 23-day, 28-day and 33-day biorhythms are exceptions to these kinds of causal influences. It would appear likely that a number of variables could restart or otherwise alter the rhythm period or cycle of each of these, just as research has confirmed this among other biological rhythms. Unusual circumstances during birth (such as a Caesarian section) might affect our start date. A trauma such as a motor vehicle accident or otherwise could cause an abrupt interference that might alter or shift the cycle. In other words, while the research may have illustrated a cycling of rhythms close to these patterns as behavior was examined over large populations; mathematical analysis of each person and each birth date illustrates too much variance to insist we are all cycling precisely the same biorhythms.

This said, there might also be entrainment influences we have yet to consider. As we discussed, our circadian cycles are significantly entrained each day to the sun's path, which tends to synchronize or tune our circadian cycles. The moon, the stars and the seasonal tilt of the earth all create potential entrainment devices for infradian rhythms. However, the precise mechanisms are larger than our scope of research. In the absence of an entrainment process such as exists with the morning light upon our pineal gland and

SCN system, it would seem likely our infradian rhythms would be distorted by the unique, personal events we each have.

Simple observation tells us that at least half the population is subject to variable but consistent infradian rhythms. Almost every female body with little variance – excepting cases of significant health disorders – between the ages of about 13 and 50, undergoes a menstrual cycle lasting between 22 and 45 days, with the median being about 28 days. In a study of 130 women at the University Of Pittsburg School Of Medicine (Creinin *et al.* 2004), the average was 29 days, with 46% having a variance of seven days and 20% cycled 14 days or less. While this is a substantial variance, the consistency of cycling among women is quite significant.

This 28- to 29-day rhythm certainly corresponds with the proposed 28-day emotional cycle of Fliess and Swoboda and others. It also appears suspicious that a woman's menstrual cycle is intimately connected with moods and physical/psychological emotional cycles. Curiously, many modern Fliess and Swoboda biorhythm proponents declare that the woman's 28-day menstrual cycle is a mere coincidence.

The female cycle begins with the flow of follicle-stimulating hormone (FSH). As named, this hormone stimulates the production of a follicle in the ovary. As the follicle develops and the ovum matures, it produces increased amounts of estrogen. As estrogen's messages are carried to receptors in the uterus, uterine cells begin to prepare the endometrium for the potential of a pregnancy. This means the endometrium begins to thicken and uterine glands elongate.

Estrogen is a complicated messenger – as most hormones are. Within a day or two before ovulation, estrogen will stimulate a spike in luteinizing hormone (LH) which converts a ruptured follicle into the corpus luteum. The corpus luteum in turn produces copious amounts of progesterone, which stimulates incremental growth among the endometrium and supporting tissues. These spikes in estrogen and progesterone also provide an inhibiting feedback response to the pituitary, slowing subsequent LH and FSH release.

Around this time – as if set by an alarm – the ovum slides into the uterus through the oviduct. Here it may or may not encounter a male sperm. If it does, fertilization may or may not occur. If not, within 2-3 solar days, the ovum will begin to deteriorate. The corpus luteum will degenerate, and estrogen and progesterone levels will fall. The endometrium also thins, and small hemorrhages poke through its lining. This causes the bleeding of menstruation. Menstruation will typically last 3-6 solar days. In Creinin, the average was 5.2 days.

During this time, new cells begin to grow within the endometrial wall. This repairs the hemorrhaged areas. As levels of estrogen and progesterone fall to their negative points on the cycle, FSH is released from the pituitary, stimulating the rhythmic cycle's repetition.

For most healthy women the flow of these hormones; the follicle and ovum growth; movement and eventual breakdown; and the subsequent repair of the system take place every month like clockwork. Again, there are significant individual differences. In a study done at Marquette University's College of Nursing (Fehring *et al.* 2006), 141 healthy women underwent testing for cycle consistency. The average of 28.9 days consisted of 95% between 22 and 36 days, while 42% had intracycle variances of more than seven days. For example, while 95% had six fertile solar days between day four and day 23, only 25% had their fertile days between day ten and day seventeen. The researchers concluded that among other parts of the intracycle, follicular phase seems to be at the root of much of the variation.

There is also significant research indicating groups of women living together or spending time in close proximity over a significant period begin to cycle to the same menstrual rhythms. This synchronization of rhythms has been the subject of research between mothers and daughters, roommates and dormitory women. In all three instances, studies have illustrated this rhythmic correlation of physical proximity between women living together (Weller and Weller 1993). In terms of occurrence, Weller *et al.* (1999) discovered that among 73 urban households with a relatively high degree of interaction, 51% menstrual synchrony occurred within families and among sisters. And 30% occurred among friends not living together. This study concluded a correlation between durable physical proximity and emotional synchrony.

As to the mechanisms of menstruation proximity, there are a number of hypotheses. Some researchers have proposed the existence of an entrainment mechanism through a type of pheromone process. Others have suggested that certain physical and social cues create a synchronized entrainment of rhythms: A sort of subconscious environmental entrainment process. This opens the strong possibility that close proximity simply allows for similar sun and light exposures.

This hypothesis is not without support. Multiple studies have confirmed menstrual dysfunction may be significantly affected by light exposure variations (Barron 2007). Disturbance also appears related to melatonin secretion – also related to light exposure. The vulnerability of the menstruation cycle to sun exposure is indicated by various psychological and physiological stressors. For example, bipolar disorder and polycystic ovary syndrome have influenced a woman's cycle in becoming more sensitive to light exposure.

What about the other half of the human population? Is the male body absent of infradian rhythms? Hardly. In 1990, Chirkova *et al.* reported in the *Laboratornoe Delo* that the serum of young healthy men revealed ten different body rhythms of different wavelengths and frequencies. Using amylase testing, several cycles were demonstrated, ranging from eight hours to one month. The authors observed nine different environmental factors – including solar entrainment – that influenced these cycles. Dr. Peter Celec and associates from Comenius University's Institute of Pathophysiology (2004) concluded that – after using an Analysis of Rhythmic Variance Test (ANORVA) on five healthy males – a strong duodecimal (12-day) rhythm of salivary estradiol levels existed in men.

Dr. Celec and his associates also used ANORVA to expose two different cycles of testosterone within the male body in a study published in 2003. Saliva was collected from 31 healthy males between the age of 20 and 22.5 years old for 75 days during the fall of 2000. Using two methods of statistical analysis to remove bias – one a moving average and the other a phase shift variance – the research unveiled both a *ciratrigintan* (monthly) and a *circavigintan* (triweekly) rhythm among testosterone production.

Pronina (1992) also found infradian rhythms among testosterone and aldosterone levels. The rhythm frequency for aldosterone was 2.5-5.5 solar days. Testosterone levels experienced two longer rhythms, one of 5-13.5 solar days, and another, stronger rhythm with a 21-day period. There was a range between age groups among the amplitudes of secretion levels. The length of the rhythms stayed consistent among different ages, however.

As was noted in the circadian discussion, daily hormone levels are destructively interfered by stress. This correlation is also found among the longer duration of the rhythms, as was discovered in a one-year study of 72 firefighters by Roy *et al.* (2003). Stress cycles were compared with cortisol and testosterone levels within these cycles. It was found that during periods of lower stress (and likely more sun exposure), cortisol levels increased and testosterone levels decreased. Inversely, during higher stress (likely with less sun exposure), cortisol levels decreased and testosterone levels increased.

Biophoton emissions – weak light pulses emanating from human cells – appear to cycle in larger infradian rhythms as well. In research by Dr. S. Cohen and Dr. Fritz Popp at the Institute of Biophysics (1997), a person was scanned daily over a period of several months for weak photon emissions. Measurements demonstrated a cycling of biophoton emissions with bi-weekly, monthly and longer cycles of intensity fluctuation. Consistent rhythms of fourteen days, one month, three months and nine months were evidenced by rising and falling photon emission levels. This demonstrated coherence between biophotons, the sun, and the release of testosterone, estrogen, melatonin, cortisol, LH and many other metabolic biochemicals flowing through the body.

This is confirmed by other research by Cohen, Popp and others illustrating that these biophoton emissions emanating from cells resonate with and entrain to the electromagnetic radiation of the sun.

By the Light of the Moon

The moon waxes and wanes with a tilted elliptical orbit around the earth, reflecting sunlight with different trajectories. It is both the moon's orbit and the reflection of the sun's light that appears to influence the moon's effects. Though controversial, a respectable body of research correlates behavior and biological metabolism with the position of the moon with respect to the sun. Thakur and

Sharma reported in the *British Medical Journal* (1984) on the incidence of crimes reported by police stations in three different Indian towns from 1978 to 1982. One town was rural, one town was urban and the other was industrial. Crime rates were higher on full moon days in all locales. Crimes were also slightly higher on new moon days.

In 1978, the *Journal of Clinical Psychiatry* (Leiber) reported a computer analysis on human aggression, homicides, suicides, traffic fatalities, and psychiatric emergency room visits in Dade County Florida. There was a significant clustering of these events around the lunar synodic cycle.

In 2000, the *British Medical Journal* published a study by Bhattacharjee *et al.* showing that of 1621 cases of animal bites to humans, incidence rose significantly during full moons.

On the other side of the 'moon' on this issue, there have also been a number of studies published indicating no correlation between extraordinary events and the full moon. One study also published in *BMJ* reported no correlation between dog bites and the full moon in 1671 cases in Australia (Chapman and Morrell 2000). A study of traffic accidents over nine years showed no correlation between the moon's cycles and traffic accidents (Laverty and Kelly 1998). Owen *et al.* (1998) showed a lack of correlation between the lunar cycle and violence in two studies. A Canary Island emergency room was studied by Núñez *et al.* in 2002. This showed a lack of correlation between emergency room entrance and the moon's cycles. Psychiatric admissions of 8,473 patients between 1993 and 2001 for a Navy Medical Center in San Diego also showed no correlation between the moon's synodic phases among psychiatric admissions (McLay *et al.* 2006).

As to the discrepancy between these results, we can propose, as others have, the possibility of a differentiation between the methods of lunar calculation. The differences between the sidereal lunar cycle and the synodic cycles are significant. While the sidereal month measures the path of the moon relative to the stars and constellations behind it to form a cycle of 27.21 days, the synodic path is measured relative to the sun's path. Because the earth is in rotation, it takes the moon about 29.5 days to cycle back to the same position when referencing the position of the sun.

Gender may also be a variant that might explain the contradictory results. In a study (Buckley *et al.*) published in a 1993 edition of the *Medical Journal of Australia,* self-poisoning of 2215 patients between 1987 and 1993 were studied. Self-poisoning among women was greatest during the new moon, at 60%. However, the result was significantly lower for men. In addition, the mean illumination of the moon was 50.63% at the time of overdose for women on average. For men it was 47.45%.

In a study by Kollerstrom and Steffert (2003) from England, four years of telephone call frequency data was compiled from a crisis call center. The new moon brought a significant increase in women callers, with a swing of 9%, and a decrease in callers by men during the new moon.

Anthropological studies have indicated a link between the new moon and menstruation among the female population (Bell and Defouw 1964). In this study, the authors also discuss the discrepancy between the various lunar cycle calculations, noting that while some have used a 30-day monthly cycle in their calculations, others have used a 28-day lunar cycle, and still others have calculated using the 29.5 synodic cycle.

Research on animals also demonstrates physiological patterns seemingly related to the moon's cycles. For example, Zimecki (2006) confirmed that lunar cycles correlate with cycles for circulating corticosterones, melatonin levels, taste perception, sleep quality, as well as pineal and hypothalamus gland activity.

No one versed in botany can deny the moon's effects upon plant growth. Farmers generally plant with phases of the moon, timed also with seasons, temperatures and moisture. These rhythmic effects of the moon on plant growth have become obvious over thousands of years of trial and error. Observation has led us to understand that the waxing moon typically stimulates plant growth as compared with a waning moon. Hence, farmers are likely to plant crops that bear aboveground fruits during the waxing moon and root crops during the waning moon. Most trees, even fruit trees – are considered root-oriented. They tend to be more vigorous when planted on the waning moon.

Studies in 1939 by Kolisko on wheat found that seeds sprouted better if they were sown during the full moon. Poor sprouting resulted from new moon plantings. Other studies have followed, confirming these findings. Northwestern Professor F. Brown found that with equal temperatures, sprouting seedlings absorb greater water at full moon. This seems to indicate that plants hold more water during the full moon as well, and consequently hold less during the new moon. Even when Brown shielded the plants from the light of the moon, they still responded to moon phase (Brown and Chow 1973).

From 1952 to 1962, biodynamic grower Maria Thun performed research on moon phases on her farm in Darmstadt, Germany. She sowed row crops systematically over sidereal-measured moon positions. She weighed crop yields using this system after each harvest. Thun found that when potatoes were planted when the moon was in Taurus, Capricorn and Virgo they had better yields than when the moon was in the other constellations. Conversely, root crops did not produce well if they were planted when the moon was in the houses of Cancer, Scorpio and Pisces. Though controversial, these results were replicated by later researchers (Kollerstrom and Staudenmaier 2001).

It appears evident that modern science has yet to fully grasp the orientation and extent of influence on behavior and biology by the various rhythms driven by the sun and moon. Thakur and Sharma mention in their analysis that the body contains at least 50-60% water; and the tidal gravitational pull upon water by the moon is evidenced by the ocean's tidal rhythms. Various environmental measurements have indicated that the moon's gravitational pull is about 23% less than its pull on full moon days.

Certainly, science's overwhelming interest to understand the potential influence heavenly bodies have upon our bodies has been cause enough for the volume of research sampled here. Many of the ancient astronomers were also leading researchers, respected mathematicians and physicians. Still, modern medicine opted to throw out this body of observational research and start from scratch. Gradually, we are accumulating the evidence that illustrates these ancient astronomers might not have been the crackpots we assumed they were. We are also hopefully learning that double-blind controlled research is not the only path towards knowledge.

Modern science currently questions how planetary bodies millions of light years away from earth could affect human activity. If we consider that simply the ability to see these stars requires the reception of the electromagnetic radiation emitted from every star, it seems at least remotely viable that the radiation of these stars may have some subtle influence. We might suppose this influence is geomagnetic, electromagnetic, and gravitational – perhaps a combination thereof.

When we look at the billions of stars on a clear night, we are often overwhelmed by the majesty and the largeness of it all. As we look with amazement at a swirling universe billions of light years away, and ponder black holes that appear to contradict the rules of matter, we have good reason for pause. The effects these bodies have upon metabolism may be subtle. Or they may be more potent than our current instruments can quantify. Perhaps the combined effects of the sun, moon and planets, together with the various thermal, atmospheric, genetic and clockwork biochemistry within the body, create a confluence of signalling systems as their combined waveforms create unique interference patterns. Perhaps the biomagnetic influences created by the relative juxtaposition of the planets amongst themselves – the ephemeris view as quantified by some of history's most respected scientists and physicians – might have some scientific credence after all.

Seasonal Solar Synchronization

Simple observation tells us that seasonal solar rhythms influence our behavior and the behavior of so many organisms. During the winter, many animals migrate or hibernate. Some humans tend to partially hibernate indoors, especially in the northern latitudes. This is evidenced by the great incidence of *seasonal affective disorder,* which appears primarily in the winter in higher latitudes among those who stay indoors. SAD – which we'll discuss later in more detail – is a sort of depression that typically occurs after a lengthy period spent indoors without natural sunlight. Research has shown that SAD is also linked to lower vitamin D production. As we will discuss in more detail later, vitamin D production is stimulated by the skin's contact with the sun's ultraviolet rays. Seasonal light reduction also results in decreased serotonin levels, as natural light stimulates the production of this mood-regulating hormone. During the winter, our body's biochemicals also stimulate an urge to eat more. We can also seasonally correlate the levels of biochemicals such as leptin, insulin, ghrelin, amylin, glucocorticoids and resistin – along with all the other energy-related biochemicals. Many of these have been linked with dysfunctions like SAD and obesity.

As the weather warms during the springtime, our bodies tend to get outside more. We tend to expose more skin to the sun. This time is also associated with romance. The 'spring fling' is experienced primarily by young adults at the peak of their reproductive years. Increased exposure to sunlight encourages increased serotonin levels. Sunlight also stimulates neurotransmitter biochemicals like dopamine that render a sense of physical well-being. We can combine these internal biochemical messengers with the exchange of a more subtle signalling system of pheromones.

The debate on whether humans exchange pheromones has recently been settled through research. This references the discovery that androstadienone from human male sweat glands increased female cortisone levels (Wyart, *et al.* 2007).

Spring is also a time of reproduction for many other species. The flowers of many plants produce pollen, which allows the male species to fertilize the female reproductive system through a complex process of joining pollen with ovule. This pollination and fertilization process leads to the production of seeds. These seeds blow into the spring and early summer winds to propagate the species. Meanwhile, many animals begin their migration to the more northern or southern latitudes (depending upon their home turf in relation to the equator) for mating in the spring. Hibernating species come out for their first meals in many months during the springtime. These behaviors synchronize with biochemicals stimulated by the changes in sunlight intensity.

During the summer, the heat comes on and activity peaks. Most trees come into full leaf, giving shade for other species in need of a respite from the hot sun. The environment tends to become drier during the summer in most northern latitudes. During this period, plant chlorophyll levels peak for maximum photosynthesis. Most animals are in peak activity periods as they hunt, forage and care for their offspring. Humans also tend to increase activity, as we will often vacation during the summer months. We head to the forests, oceans, or lakes for a natural escape into the sun.

During the fall as the sun retreats to other latitudes, organisms prepare for the retreat of the sun. Trees begin to drop their leaves, preparing for another round of rhythmic dormancy. Animals begin their rhythmic migration to warmer climates. School begins, and humans rhythmically return to the partial hibernation of indoor activities.

These seasonal cycles resonate with the rhythmicity of the sun's relative path through our skies. Activity cycles with the off-centered rotation of the earth, which repositions the sun to create the cyclic variation of daylight and solar exposure. Increased daylight accompanies a greater spectrum of radiation: More ultraviolet light, visible light and infrared radiation. With this increase in waveform spectrum comes an increase in energy levels. Reproduction is stimulated. Activity is stimulated. During the negative cycle, decreased daylight and lower temperatures decrease energy levels, decrease reproduction and lower activity. Each cycle creates a balance contributing to the wellness of the organism. Without the combination of the positive and negative rhythms of the sun's seasonal cycles, exhaustion or complete inactivity would result.

The ancient science of *Ayurveda* correlated and classified six seasons of the year with the clockwork rhythms of the body. In the northern latitudes, the late winter season (mid-January to mid-March in the northern latitudes) is known as the *sishira* portion of the year. During this time, there is a predominance of cold and wet weather. The *vasanta* season, lasting from mid-March to mid-May, is the classic spring season. The *grishma* period is the early summer season, until mid-July. The next season is *varsha*, or the rainy season, which in Asia and many tropical areas lasts until mid-September. The *sharat* season is the typical autumn season, lasting until mid-November, and the *hemant* season is the colder early winter season. Each season is connected with predominant lifestyle activities, types of foods and general lifestyle choices in *Ayurveda*. Each is connected to a combination of the qualities of *kapha, vata* or *pitta*.

In *Ayurveda,* each season is also accompanied by particular taste associations as well. The wet winter season is associated with bitter taste, while the spring is associated with astringent taste. The summer is associated with hot taste, the rainy season associated with sour taste, the autumn associated with salty taste and the winter associated with sweet taste. Here are some other seasonal tendencies detailed in the ancient science of *Ayurveda*:

Wet winter: digestive activity increases and *kapha* is increased. Heavier foods are eaten with more wheat and dairy products. Sweet, sour and fatty foods are also typically increased. Foods and clothing are thicker and warmer. Increased exposure to fire is recommended. Increased exercise is recommended. Massage is oily.

Spring season: Excess *kapha* is cleansed during the spring but digestion is slowed. Therefore, light and easily digested food is recommended. Yogurts and other fermented foods are recommended. Fruits and vegetables to increase detoxification are suggested. Avoiding sour, sweet and fatty foods is suggested. Massage is dry.

Early summer season: As *kapha* is cleansed, *pitta* begins. Light foods are continued, but sweet and fatty foods are added. Cold water and fruits are recommended. Cold baths, cool places, light clothing are all suggested. Chandan paste is recommended for body anointing.

Late summer: In rainy areas, digestion is worsened as *kapha* and *pitta* compete in the humidity. In dry regions, *pitta* increases with some *vata* tendencies building late. Cooling foods are recommended, together with cool baths and plenty of swimming. Fruits and light foods are suggested, together with pulses and yogurt drinks.

Autumn/Early winter: The dryness of autumn and the dry cold of early winter aggravate the *vata* element – known for coldness and dryness. Therefore, recommended foods are astringent or sweet. Warm foods are suggested. Grains are good and food should be low in oil. Warm oil massages are increased.

Many of these recommendations – such as light foods in the summer – are logical responses to environmental conditions. Still, many people will not follow these natural behavior rhythms because of stress or other habits. Like many ancient regimens, the ancient Ayurvedic system is a general guide for appropriate rhythmic behavior, in an attempt to live more harmonically with our environment. According to *Ayurveda*, atypical habits can interfere with our body's normal cycling through the seasons. The influences of each season also depend upon which characteristics dominate in each body type. A person with a predominantly *pitta* physical body and consciousness might be aggravated more by the hot weather than a person who is dryer and more *vatic*, for example. The *vatic* person would be more susceptible to variances between the suggested seasonal diets, on the other hand. Meanwhile a *kapha* type may be comfortable during the winter months as they cozy up to plenty of food and warmth. However, the *kapha* type may also be subject to increased mucus and disease due to an excess of these activities, unless they detoxify properly, according to *Ayurveda*.

Unique seasonal activities are also supported by science. Recent research unveils how seasonal patterns affect birth. In one study of more than 75,000 births in a Pittsburgh hospital between 1995 and 2004, pre-term deliveries were 25% less likely for summer and fall conception than for winter conception (Bodnar and Simhan 2007). In an Indiana University School of Medicine (Tweed 2007) study of 1,667,391 Indiana students between third and tenth grade, it was found that students conceived between June and August had the lowest test scores in math and language. A number of theories have been proposed to explain these seasonal differences. Regardless, the benefits for seasonal behavior are undeniable.

Our bodies also pass through 'seasons' as they age. According to *Ayurveda,* each person's unique *dosha* tends to evolve with each season of the body's lifespan. During childhood, growth and development predominates. As a result, this period is said to be the *kapha* period, where mucus and anabolism prevails. During young adulthood through adulthood, *pitta* is said to prevail. During this period sexual activity peaks, metabolism peaks, family life prevails and core body temperature heightens. During this period, the person will be less tolerant to hot weather. Then, in the body's elderly years, *vata* tendencies become greater. The body becomes dryer, metabolism slows (catabolism), and a period of slow emotional detachment should begin. During this time, the body tends to tolerate heat more – especially dry heat. With each passing *dosha* season, certain tastes predominate, changing over time with learning. Children usually avoid spicy or salty foods but crave cold, sweet and sour foods. Adults tend to be attracted to detoxifying spicy, hot, and salty foods as they age. The elderly tend to appreciate warm foods with increasingly sweet and bitter tastes as their metabolism slows and emotion levels out.

The ancient Chinese codification system also connects rhythmic cycles to the passing of years. According to ancient Chinese science, one macro cycle is 60-years long, consisting of five cycles of twelve years. These twelve-year cycles are named after animals because each has a distinct predominating quality. Each year also has an attribute of either *yin* or *yang* as that cycle is considered to have a behavioral effect. Thus, each year will be distinguished as either *yin* or *yang*, one of the five elements, and one of the animal-like qualities. Recommended activities are coordinated with each of these cycles. The traditional Chinese calendar has a number of other characteristics in tune with solar rhythms. The months are paced by lunar periods, and the year is calculated using a combination of solar year and lunar year.

Solar Rhythm Strategies

* **Biorhythm cycles:** While it is unlikely that our bodies all cycle with the same periods, there is a solid basis for connecting our activities with solar rhythms. Our physiology, metabolism and cognitive abilities are certainly affected by the sun's activity. Calculating our potential classic biorhythm cycles and testing whether these cycles correspond to our periodic ups and downs (and critical days) may reveal at the very least, some of our own unique rhythms. Should we uncover our unique cycles, we might consider timing extraordinary events with non-critical days.

* **Outdoor activities:** Spending a significant amount of time outside everyday is essential to just about every part of our metabolism. Should we not take part in our external environment, we will be missing the effects of many of the sun's effective entrainment of our body's rhythms. This will affect our sleep and our health in negative ways. Walking, exercising, gardening and/or playing outside are the best activities. Those of us who stay huddled indoors are most likely surrounded by electronics. This means that our

rhythms are cycling with the electromagnetic frequencies of our televisions, computers, video games, stereos and other appliances. We might consider scheduling electronics use around our solar schedule rather than the inverse. This means turning off the computer or television during certain parts of the day and simply going outside.

* **Time outside:** It may not be practical to break away from our indoor work environment to spend the rest of the day outside. Optimally, at least 1-2 hours outside a day are recommended. For the busy working person, a useful strategy would be to spend 15-20 minutes outside during the morning (around sunrise would be best, but any part of the morning will help) and the period prior to and just following sunset (or some part of the late afternoon) These two periods help entrain and resynchronize the body's cycles to nature's cycles.

* **Reducing stress:** If done timely and daily, morning and evening sun exposure will also reduce our stress levels. Whenever we are particularly stressed, we can make an effort to step outside or at least watch the sunset or sunrise from a window. It is amazing how easily the stresses seem to fall away with the transitional sun exposure of the sunset and sunrise.

* **Improving digestion:** Eating with the sun's cycles is critical to proper digestion. Our gastrin, enzyme and bile salt release is entrained not just to the smell of food. It is also entrained to the sun. Our probiotic systems are also entrained to the physical changes that take place due to exposure to the sun. It is best to try to eat early in the day following sunrise, mid-day when the sun is highest, and just following sunset. Our digestive cycles are primed with the cortisol and melatonin release cycles. The digestive tracts of human beings have been entrained to the sun's cycles for thousands of years.

* **Food choices:** Our food choices complement the timing of our meals. A morning meal with fiber and fruit and

maybe some nuts and dairy if tolerated will stimulate a gradual glycemic response while stimulating energy from the protein. A mid-day lunch with grains and vegetables will balance metabolism with cortisol levels. A post-sunset evening meal of salad, fibrous grains and/or beans with dairy if tolerated and maybe some fruit dessert will encourage healthy melatonin levels later in the evening. Mid-meal snacks of fruit or nuts help close the glycemic gap during high-energy days.

* **Improving sleep quality:** Sleeping is best done in complete darkness or under the stars. Research illustrates that sleep quality is decreased after sunrise and during daylight hours. Even the smallest electric night light can lower our levels of melatonin and reduce sleep quality. Our body cycles melatonin highest at night and our cortisol levels cycle lowest at night. This is part of nature's design. Our bodies will relax more at night, allowing all the cells to recycle and rejuvenate as the immune system kicks into high gear.

* **Evening light:** Into the evening, our lights should slowly be lowered as the night proceeds, to help advance our melatonin levels. Our computer and TV use should slow down as we get closer to bedtime. Bright bathroom lights are discouraged during the pre-bedtime period. A bright light will immediately stimulate our pineal gland, which will increase cortisol levels and slow down melatonin levels. This will increase our risk of not falling asleep.

* **Working at night:** Working during the evening when melatonin levels are higher confuses the body's metabolism. This confusion will stimulate the flow of adrenaline and cortisol, which increase body temperature, stimulate stress response, reduce relaxation, defer immune response and many others.

* **Exercise:** Exercising in the evening will increase body core temperature, delaying the production of melatonin, which helps our bodies relax and get to sleep. Exercise is best done in the morning or afternoon, preferably outside.

* **Rhythmic water consumption:** Drinking 2-3 cups of room-temperature water first thing in the morning helps to hydrate the body after a night of dehydrated sleeping (as water drank at night will reduce sleep quality with nighttime urination). Daytime water intake of ten or so glasses per day are recommended *between meals* – as absorption is more efficient on an empty stomach. Drinking daily water at the same times each day is recommended to maximize absorption and cellular hydration.

* **Moon planning:** Working with the moon's rhythms can help us in a variety of ways. Activities requiring more creativity, planning and focus can be done with the new moon. Activities requiring more stamina, endurance or peak performance can be planned around the full moon. Gardening or farming can certainly be planned around the moon's cycles as we have discussed. In many ways, our lives can be planned out and arranged as we might arrange a garden. Root-oriented plants are similar to activities that develop our grounding and internal growth. These are better begun during the waning moon. Activities intended for external success or productivity are better begun with the waxing moon.

* **Seasonal behavior:** Seasonal activities are also important to maximize health and energy. Vacationing around the same time every year is recommended. More time outside during the summer should balance reduced daylight hours during the winter. Morning and late afternoon-evening daylight hours are recommended during the summer.

* **Seasonal sun timing:** We've already established that sunrise and sunset are minimum times to be outside. During the wintertime, we should plan other outdoor activities during the mid-day or afternoon to maximize our vitamin D production (we'll discuss the in more detail later). During the summer, morning and late afternoon sun are best to reduce the risk of sunburn.

* **Seasonal food choices:** Lighter foods with more fruits and vegetables are appropriate in the summer, while more grains, beans and fattier foods are more appropriate for the fall and winter.

* **Daylight savings:** This is an outdated and unhealthy program. The change in the clocks related to daylight savings time can cause confusion to the body and its seasonal and daily cycling with the sun. Following the time change, care should be taken to maintain the same eating and sleeping solar times if possible. At least for a while. Gradually, we can alter our sleeping and eating schedules to the new time.

* **Jet lag strategies:** When traveling, pay close attention to the body's solar clock with respect to light exposure. *To reduce jet lag at our destination:* During the day of travel, delay daylight exposure to the destination's solar times on the day of travel. When at the destination, find a mid-way point between the sunset solar time of departure location and destination location, and maintain that solar daylight exposure for that day (of arrival). Then the next day, increase morning daylight exposure halfway towards the destination's solar time, and be outside at the destination at sunset. The next day, match both the morning and evening solar daylight exposure by being outside during or close to both times (sunrise and sunset). To simulate darkness, avoid bright lights, stay inside and wear dark sunglasses. To maximize daylight exposure, keep sunglasses off and be outside as much as possible. *Example: Say you are traveling from California to New York. The solar time difference is three hours. During the day of travel, wear sunglasses and avoid the sun until 9 a.m. (assuming 6 a.m. sunrise). On the first day after arrival in New York, be outside until 5:30 p.m. (assuming a 7pm sunset). The next morning, keep shades down and/or sunglasses on until 7:30 a.m. Then go outside into the daylight. Spend as much time outside in the daylight as possible. That evening, stay or be outside until the sunset at 7 p.m. The next morning, awake with the sunrise and go outside into the daylight with no sunglasses. That evening, try to be outside at or around sunset. Your body clock should now be set to current time.*

Chapter Two

The Biomagnetic Sun

In addition to the sun's pervasive rhythmic influences over our metabolism, we find growing evidence of its significant biomagnetic effects. Though sunspots and solar storms were observed by many over the centuries, Galileo is given credit for making the first correct interpretation of sunspots on the sun's surface. Then in the early nineteenth century, astronomers began to notice a periodic cycling of sunspot activity. This led to further correlation between solar storm activity and environmental changes. Later, behavioral effects were recognized. Over the years, scientists have correlated birth rates, ice ages, wars, epidemics and other events with the sun's solar storm activity.

Solar flares and subsequent proton storms provide an interactive relationship between the sun and its production of thermal radiation. Cyclical solar flares erupt on the surface of the sun, sending various forms of radiation such as x-ray flares and protons into its immediate atmosphere. Some of these flares eject out in *coronal masses*, which appear like tentacles reaching out into space. These events hurl electromagnetic waves through the solar system. Their projections can create damage for orbiting vehicles and can penetrate the earth's atmosphere, causing power outages and radio blackouts.

Solar storms also create a shield effect for the earth. The biomagnetic fields created by solar storms prevent damaging cosmic rays from intruding upon the earth's biosphere. This was discovered recently as scientists correlated carbon-14 levels in trees and the atmosphere (through rock and ice readings) with solar storm activity. Periods of higher solar storm activity were met with reduced carbon-14 levels. This indicated a protective effect from the sun. It also meant that solar storm activity has also coincided with global cooling and heating trends.

In 1843, German astronomer Samuel Schwabe first documented his observations of solar activity, noting that sunspot activity appeared to be periodic. Over many years of subsequent analysis by astrophysicists, it has been determined that sunspot cycles range from 9 years to 14 years, with an average of 11.1 years. Within this obvious cyclical behavior, astronomers also noticed other cycles occurring within the period of each cycle. Advances in monitoring technology revealed these explosions – called solar flares – move cyclically with respect to their intensity. When sunspot and solar flare activity are graphed over more than a century, a harmonic butterfly-shaped waveform is revealed.

In the 1950s, the American astronomer Dr. Harold Babcock detailed the magnetic field distribution on the sun's surface. Using his invention, the *solar magnetograph,* Dr. Babcock determined that the sun reverses magnetic polarity on a periodic basis. He also found that stars also emit unique magnetic fields.

The correlation between human behavior and solar cycles is due largely to the research of Russian scientist Alexander Chizhevsky. Chizevsky is also known for his groundbreaking research discovering the properties of ionized air during the earlier part of the twentieth century.

In the early 1920s, Chizhevsky analyzed the timing of wars, battles, riots, and revolutions among the histories of 72 countries from 500 BCE to 1922. He discovered that 80% of these critical events took place close to a sunspot activity peak. In an attempt to explain the data, Chizhevsky proposed that strong magnetic fields might be emanating from these intense solar storms. He suggested that magnetic influences from solar storms could trigger mass behavior changes among large populations simultaneously. These magnetic stimulatory effects, he thought, could affect mental propensities, predisposing aggressive or violent behavior.

Chizhevsky's studies demonstrated similar patterns between solar sunspot cycles and mortality rates caused by epidemics and spikes in births. The relevance and conclusions from his research have recently received confirmation in research by Musaev *et al.* (2007), which studied demographic data together with infectious disease mortality between 1930 and 2000. Disease and mortality statistics related to cardiovascular, neurological, oncological, bronchi-pulmonary, and infectious pandemics were compared. The data indicated a clear relationship between these pathology statistics and solar storm activity cycles.

This research was considered novel and controversial during Chizhevsky's lifetime. However, continued research over the decades since Chizhevsky has confirmed a number of significant

effects caused by what is now referred to as *geomagnetism* upon behavior and disease.

Recent research has uncovered many pathological effects resulting from the geomagnetic influence of auroras, sunspots and solar
storms. The Cardiology department of Israel's Rabin Medical Center (Stoupel *et al.* 2007) studied the occurrence of acute myocardial
infarction together with the timing and measurement of solar activity. They differentiated the effects of higher cosmic ray activity
from periods of higher geomagnetic activity (sunspots and solar
flares). This study found myocardial infarction rates inversely correlated with monthly solar activity, and positively correlated with
increased cosmic ray activity. Low geomagnetic activity days and
higher cosmic ray days were both separately linked with significantly
greater rates of fatalities due to myocardial infarction.

Marasanov and Matveev also reported in 2007 that among lung
cancer patients having surgery, complications occurred more significantly during geomagnetic solar storm periods than during
geomagnetic "quiet" days.

In 2006, Stoupel *et al.* calculated immune system strength by
measuring IgG, IgM, IgA, lupus anti-coagulant, clotting time and
autoantibody blood levels of subjects. These levels were correlated
with periods and strengths of solar activity as measured by the U.S.
National Geophysical Data Center. This research found that immune system biomarker levels significantly decrease with solar
geomagnetic activity.

Stoupel's research confirmed studies done at Canada's Lauren-
tian University (Kinoshameg and Persinger 2004) which concluded
that rats exposed to induced geomagnetic activity suffered immunosuppression, resulting in higher rates of infection.

In 2006, Yeung analyzed pandemic influenza outbreaks from
1700 A.D. to 2000 A.D. Significant correlations were found between
outbreak periods and sunspot cycles.

Vaquero and Gallego (2007) confirmed the connection between
immunosuppression, infectious outbreaks, and sunspot cycles in
research studying pandemic influenza A.

A 2006 study from researchers from Kyoto University in Japan
(Otsu *et al.*) reported that a strong correlation existed between sunspot activity, unemployment rates and suicides between 1971 and

2001. Both unemployment and suicides were inversely proportional to sunspot rhythmic periods.

Another study from 2006 (Davis and Lowell) using the birth dates of 237,000 humans found a positive correlation between the births of children with genetic mental diseases like schizophrenia and bipolar disorder with solar activity. They also found similar correlations between solar activity cycles and 'genetic' diseases like multiple sclerosis and rheumatoid arthritis. These diseases were also closely correlated with being born in a particular season.

In another study done in Israel (Stoupel et al. 2006), 339,252 newborn births over a period of seven years were compared to monthly cosmic ray and solar activity. Significantly more babies were born of both genders during higher cosmic ray periods. In other words, fewer newborns were born during high solar activity periods as compared with low or non-solar activity periods.

The Rabin Medical Center (Stoupel et al. 2005) also studied Down syndrome cases among 1,108,449 births together with solar activity. With 1,310 total cases of Down syndrome in the data, a significant inverse relationship between solar activity occurred (r=-0.78). In other words, Down syndrome – long considered a genetic defect – occurs more often during the periods between solar activity, and less often during periods of solar activity.

Researchers at the Universidad de Chile's Clinica Psiquiatrica Universitaria (Ivanovic-Zuvic et al.) presented a study in 2005 that compared increased hospitalizations of depressive patients and manic patients to solar activity periods. In this study, depressive hospitalizations correlated with periods of lower solar activity, while manic hospitalizations positively correlated with higher solar activity periods.

A study at the Augusta Mental Health Institute in Maine (Davis and Lowell 2004) established that excessive ultraviolet radiation from the sun combined with solar flare cycles correlated positively with mental illnesses resulting from DNA damage.

It also appears from research as reported by Davis and Lowell (2004) that human lifespan correlates with solar activity. From this research, chaotic solar cycles (as opposed to typical cycles) coincide with increases in mutagenic DNA effects. Further exploration into lifespan and birthdates around solar cycles found disrupted solar cycles correlating positively with shorter lifespan.

In an Australian study (Berk *et al.* 2006) of suicides between 1968 and 2002, both seasonal and geomagnetic solar storm activity were investigated using 51,845 male and 16,327 female suicides. Suicides among females significantly increased in the autumn, concurrent with increased geomagnetic storm activity. Suicides were lowest during autumn for males and lowest during the summer for females. The average number of suicides for both males and females were the greatest during the spring.

This connection of seasonal and geomagnetic activity with suicide was also confirmed in research on 27,469 Finnish suicide cases between 1979 and 1999 by Partonen *et al.* (2004).

As Kamide (2005) commented in his paper in *Biomedical Pharmacotherapy*: *"The earth is located within the solar atmosphere."*

Body Magnetic

Our physical bodies permeate with magnetism. Every ion, every atom, every molecule, every cell and every organ pulses with magnetic fusion. Our bodies and the living organisms around us and inside of us are, in fact, magnetic by nature.

Magnets were named after the lodestone – a rock found by the Greeks in the province of Magnesia. This was a curious stone, and it was observed by early Greek physicians to have healing properties. The Greek philosopher-physician Aristophanes explored this mysterious rock for many years. Hippocrates utilized the magnet for many treatments. Chinese medicine physicians also used magnets for healing centuries earlier. Over the centuries, texts show that everything from heart disease to gout was treated with magnets in Chinese, Greek, medieval, and Ayurvedic therapies.

In 1175, English monk Alexander Neckam experimented with and eventually described how a magnet could be used in a compass. In 1269, Petrus Peregrinus de Marincourt described the pivot compass. William Gilbert's sixteenth century *De Magnete* described many other uses for the magnet, and described the pointing of a magnetized needle to not only the north direction of the compass but also downward. From this, he proposed that the earth must have a *"magnetic soul."*

The realization of magnetism's inter-relationship with electricity donned on Michael Faraday in 1831 when he coiled wire around an iron ring and demonstrated induction by passing a magnet through the ring. Faraday followed these demonstrations by calculating the relationships and proclaiming four formulas as the basis for what is now known as the *Field theory*. Faraday's proposals for a combined electromagnetic effect were not well received, however. As many discoveries are, they were not accepted for many years.

The famous homopolar generator followed these theories. The electric generator is in use even today as the primary method of advancing direct current through a circuit – the most basic form of electrical generation – still referred to as induction. Should it be directed through a circulating magnetic disk, the induction begins to alternate with the rotation. This phenomenon is often called *Faraday's disc*.

Within a few years of Faraday's work, Heinrich Ruhmkorff developed a higher-voltage pulse from DC current. The *Ruhmkorff coil* consisted of copper wires coiled around an iron core – very similar to Faraday's disk. As a DC current was passed through one of his coils, current potential increased. When the pulse was shorted or interrupted, the immediate magnetic field decrease drove the voltage to jump into high gear onto the second coil. This could be arced out to an outlet line, producing a large spike in the voltage with a pulsed, alternating flow of current.

Various demonstrations of these properties led to a maturity of the notion that Faraday initially proposed – the concept that electricity and magnetism were inter-connected: A change to one provoked a change in the other. While the notion of light and electricity as combined electromagnetic vectors was proposed by Faraday some thirty years prior, scientific acceptance followed the writings of Scot James Maxwell in the 1860s. Maxwell not only proposed the cooperating nature of electricity and magnetic fields, but also proposed that sunlight was a combination of these two fields pulsing through space.

The distribution of this strange alternating current called electricity took a big leap when physicist and fire alarm designer William Stanley conjured a crude AC electrical installation at a New York Fifth Avenue store. Prior to that, the distribution of direct current was dominated by the technical and marketing savvy of Thomas Edison.

Polarity is the key ingredient of magnetism, and shifting polarity is a driver of alternating current. In any organism, the polarity of the biomolecules and atoms making up the living cells are arranged in such a way that the poles of each molecule balance each other. This is primarily because negative and positive poles tend to attract each other. Solid structures have latticed patterns founded upon this polarity balance. This balance creates stability between the intercellular organelles, the inner and outer cell membranes, organ tissues, and other components of the body.

Most biomolecules are either *paramagnetic* (attracted to a magnet) or *diamagnetic* (repelled by a magnet), depending upon which way their polarity balance is trending. In a lodestone or ferro-magnet, however, there is a little less balance in the structure. Groupings of magnetic atoms align together with their poles pointing in one direction or another. These aligned groupings tend to overwhelm unaligned atoms of the substance, rendering a large section (oftentimes one end) polar in one direction or another. The ability to attract or repel other substances works via this strong polarity on one side of the magnet. As a result, the groupings of polarity will reorganize themselves on one side and another group will form with the opposite polarity on the other side. The strength of a field created by this polarity is typically measured in gauss or Teslas. A Tesla is 10,000 gauss.

When an electronic pulse moves through a magnetic field, the electron flow will be drawn either away from or towards the magnet, depending upon the polarity. The forward motion of the electronic current creates an arc. This arc is a representation or by-product of angular momentum. As electronic currents and magnetic fields interact together in nature, this angular momentum effect creates a display of synchronized duality.

The dynamics of magnetic induction between the sun and the earth also creates a pathway for the magnetic arc.

In a simple sense, if we were to consider the trajectory of an arrow shot upwards, it would continue in a straight line until it was acted upon by another force. Since an arrow's path typically curves upward, arcs, and then curves downward, we can say that the force of gravity was acting in a direction opposing the (upward) direction of the arrow. As we look at the perfect arc of the arrow as it heads back to earth, we can understand the direction of the force of gravity. In the same way, the pulsing of electromagnetic waves from the sun creates an arcing of magnetism perpendicular to the flow of the pulse direction.

The earth is a giant magnet, and so are all living organisms. Geologists propose that the earth is magnetic due to the motion of magnetic metals within the surface – a sort of liquefied magnetic core. The concept of a core in motion stems from the fact that the earth's magnetic fields are not static, but are changing. Findings from mountain and desert core samples show that the earth's magnetic north and south poles have varied from the current poles over the past few million years. The magnetic North Pole is now near Bathurst Island – equidistant from the north geographic pole and the Canada's Arctic Circle. The magnetic South Pole is located close to Hobart, Tasmania. In the late sixteenth century, William Gilbert measured the north magnetic declination at 10 degrees east. By the early nineteenth century, it was 25 degrees west. Now the north magnetic pole lies about 6 degrees west. The magnetic north pole is by no means static.

Core samples with magnetometer readings have confirmed that the earth's magnetic flow has maintained the same approximate direction over the past 700,000 years. Before that, the magnetic field direction of the earth changed a number of times. More than once, the poles have completely reversed. Several times in the planet's history, the earth's major magnetic field has traveled from east to west. Measurements are now illustrating that there is an overall weakening of the magnetic field – some 16% since 1670. This indicates that there is a reversal or another abrupt change in progress. Some estimate a complete phase change – or reversal – -could come as soon as 2000 years from now.

The moving core theory is not the only theory that attempts to explain the moving of magnetic direction. Some have proposed magnetic direction changes are caused by the motion of magnetic field loops circulating from east to west within the earth's interior. This rhythmic field looping has been compared to the rotating magnetism apparent between each side of a bar magnet as it changes polarity. Still others have proposed that an impact from a large meteor might be strong enough to change the earth's magnetic field. The emerging possibility is that the sun's rhythmic biomagnetic fields are created by solar storms. Quite certainly, the sun's solar storms are a contributing factor.

Research on animal migration has confirmed that migratory movement is directly related to the earth's magnetic fields. After years of debate and speculation, 1974 studies at Cornell University disclosed migration's link to magnetism. Researchers tied magnets on bird's heads and let them fly. The birds became disoriented. They had little or no ability for flight navigation until the magnets were taken off. Further testing with birds and other migrating species such as lobsters have since confirmed that all migrating organisms find their direction using tiny magnetic elements within certain cells. These coordinate their subtle polarities in the direction of travel. They relate to certain nerve cells that contain magnetite metals. These metals orient with the earth's polarity to guide the migratory path – much the same way a compass might be used by a ship's navigator to steer a course over the sea.

The research of Heyers *et al.* (2007) has revealed the likelihood that birds actually see the geomagnetic field. Experimental neuronal tracing within the eyes and forebrain of migratory birds have indicated highly active rhythmic impulses, consistent with visual signal pathways during magnetic compass bearing. *Crypotochromes* found in the neurons of the eye and in the forebrain appear to confirm this hypothesis.

Amazingly, magnetic cells have also been found in the smallest of species. Magnetic components have been found even within bacteria, for example. Many bacteria could very well be compared to bar magnets, in fact. Tiny pieces of magnetite material will line up within the center of a bacterium – approximating a rudimentary spine. This observation has led some researchers to speculate that the human spine is also magnetic. This theory seems to be supported by the various clinical successes with magnetic spinal therapy. Indeed, researchers have recently discovered magnetic molecules such as iron oxide within certain human brain and spinal nerve cells. Thus, we might conclude that our bodies also contain little magnetic compasses.

The concept of magnetism within the human physiology arose again as late-nineteenth century Julius Bernstein proposed that nerve impulses transferred through polarization. This *membrane polarization* model became the basis for the later conclusive research of Otto Loewi in the early 1920s, which led to his 1936 Nobel Prize for synaptic transmission. Loewi's experiment – which apparently occurred to him during a dream – was to extract two frog hearts and retain each in a separate bath of saline. Some of the solution surrounding the faster heartbeat was extracted and put into the bath of the other heart. This made the other heart beat faster. The experiment effectively provided the evidence for biochemical synaptic transmission.

The polarity exchange between ions and biochemicals is unmistakably magnetic. Magnetism is, after all, a polarity issue of ions or atoms aligning in one direction or another. The irrefutable link between magnetism and biological response has been confirmed by study and clinical application during the last half of the twentieth century, as the existence of ion channels has been clarified.

Furthermore, the link between intention and magnetism has become evident. This was illustrated by Dr. Grad's research at Canada's McGill University in the late 1950s and early 1960s, when growth rates of barley sprouts were stimulated by the focused intentions of particularly gifted individuals. Further studies indicated these growth rate effects were similar to the influence magnetism has on plant growth.

The central subject of these investigations was a Hungarian refugee named Oskar Estebany, who appeared to be able to exert intentional effects with his hands. A number of tests confirmed that magnetism was involved in Mr. Estebany's abilities. In one, Dr. Justa Smith at the Rosary Hill College (1973) compared Mr. Estebany's ability to increase enzyme reaction rates with those of magnetic field emissions. After Mr. Estebany affected an increase in reactivity among enzyme reaction rates, Dr. Smith applied magnetic fields and compared the rates. It turned out that the increased growth caused by Mr. Estebany precisely matched the growth caused by a 13,000 gauss magnetic field. The results indicated that somehow, intention could affect magnetic polarity.

Dr. Smith had spent a number of years studying these effects prior to and after her tests with Mr. Estebany. She authored a book on the topic – *Effect of Magnetic Fields on Enzyme Reactivity* (1969). While this research was considered radical at that time, other scientists soon confirmed her findings. In the 1990s, a flurry of research was published from around the world showing magnetic fields in the 2,500-10,000 gauss range affecting reaction rates of various enzymatic reactions. By 1996, more than fifty different enzyme reactions were found to be influenced by magnetic fields. In two linked studies by University of Utah's Charles Grissom, (1993, 1996), single-beam UV-to-visible spectrum and rapid-scanning spectrophotometers with electromagnets built in were applied to two different cobalamine (B12) enzymes. One enzyme (ethanolamine ammonia lyase) had significantly different reaction rates in response to magnetic fields, while the other enzyme (methylmalonyl CoA mutase) had no apparent response. It could thus be concluded that some biochemical processes are sensitive to magnetic field influence and others are not. This effect is still mysterious, but it has become increasingly evident that within the body lie drivers of magnetic fields.

There have been a number of controlled studies showing that major body centers respond to magnetic stimulation. Amassian *et al.* (1989) stimulated the motor cortex with a focal magnetic coil, which rendered movement to paralyzed appendages. Maccabee *et al.* (1991) stimulated almost the entire nervous system with a magnetic coil. This particular stimulation instigated responses from the distal peripheral nerve, the nerve root, the cranial nerve, the motor cortex, the premotor cortex, the frontal motor areas related to speech, and other nerve centers.

Dr. Howard Friedman and Dr. Robert Becker studied human behavior and magnetic fields in the early 1960s. They found *extremely low frequencies* (ELF) such as .1 or .2 Hz affected volunteer reaction times (Becker 1985). This paralleled work by Dr. Norbert Weiner and Dr. James Hamer with low-intensity fields, seen as "driving" waveforms already existing in the body. Spaniard Dr. Jose Delgado's research illustrated that low intensity ELF magnetic fields could influence sleep and manic behavior among monkeys. Furthermore, a substantial amount of evidence demonstrates that magnetic fields generated from power lines and transformers can modulate physiology. This has been especially noticeable in power line and transformer effects upon plants. Research linking cancer and power lines has been controversial. Still, enough evidence enables a conclusion that magnetic fields can alter certain physiological processes, as we'll discuss in more detail later.

The magnetic nature of the body is revealed through *nuclear magnetic resonance* (NMR). Its application of *magnetic resonance imaging* (MRI) is now one of the more useful diagnostic machines used in medicine when a true cross-sectional analysis of the body is required. The NMR scan is performed on the human body by surrounding the body with strong magnetic fields. These fields polarize the hydrogen (H+) proton ions in water (as the body is mostly water). As these ions' north poles align, they emit a particular frequency. Radio beams positioned around the body (tuned to this frequency) give detectors a cross-sectional scan of the body via these polarized ions. The body is guided underneath magnetic fields ranging from about 5000 to 20,000 gauss (the earth's magnetic field is about .5 gauss). As the polarity-altered hydrogen protons become excited with radio signals, a computer calculates the water content differences to form an image of the body. Were it not for the magnetic nature of the body's molecules, these three-dimensional images would not be possible.

Ironically, humankind now utilizes magnetization as our central means for information storage. We magnetize various types of oxide films with special magnetic heads. Our computer hard drives, CD players, DVD players, and tape recorders all use magnetic heads to store information as polar molecules. As we increasingly move away from the paper society, we find our society beholden to these fleeting magnetic moments of data storage. One large magnetic pulse from the sun – as was illustrated in 1989 with a nine hour Quebec blackout from a large solar flare – could easily wipe out gigantic chunks of critical data across our society – a magnetic tsunami of sorts.

Recent discoveries involving magnets and data include the finding of *single molecule magnets*. Professor George Christou and his research group at Indiana University have isolated several of these SSMs, allowing even more data can be recorded onto magnetic media. In the late 1990s, IBM accomplished a new record for hard-drive magnetic data storage, obtaining three gigabits – or three billion bits – of data storage onto one square centimeter of area of cobalt magnetic material. The SMM technology has since enabled the expansion of capacity to 30,000 billion bits – 10,000 times the IBM record (Soler *et al.* 2000).

In considering our use of magnetized information, the magnetic material within brain cells, the pulsing of magnetically driven brain waves, and the magnetic nature of migratory travel, we can safely conclude several mechanisms exist for the influence of geomagnetic emissions from the sun and its solar storm activity upon our behavior, cognition and health.

Earthly Magnetism

There is also good reason to believe that the earth's physiology is intimately connected with the geomagnetic flows from the sun. This becomes especially apparent when considering the moon's relative effects upon the planet.

In order for a solar eclipse to take place, the new moon and the sun have to be within one degree of the same declination. Due to the massive difference in the two bodies, this also means the moon must be positioned within the earth's orbit in such a way that blocks the sun's electromagnetic flows to a significant degree. A lunar eclipse, in contrast, takes place when the moon moves into the earth's shadow. This requires both the sun and moon to be exactly opposite each other with the earth in the middle.

The solar eclipse tends to affect the side of the earth where it shows itself more fully, simply because the two bodies are lined up with that side opposing the sun. This pulls the waters of the earth towards the moon. This affect is evident in the changing of tides.

For thousands of years, the period around the eclipse of the new moon has been associated with earthquakes. The Greeks documented this cycle. Early Greek writers Thucydides and Phlegon documented this link between earthquakes and new moon eclipses. Prior to that, Egyptian and Vedic cultures noted this trend. Over the past two decades, a number of seismology researchers have also proposed this link. A rash of recent quakes has also followed this trend. The San Francisco quake of 1989, the 1999

Turkish quake, the Sumatra earthquake and the tsunami of 2004 all occurred shortly before or after a solar eclipse. The Italian Physical Society published a study (Palumbo 1989) linking various other earthquakes to lunar cycles as well.

While this theory remains unproven, earthquakes appear to be related to the lunar-solar cycles somehow. In 2004, UCLA's Department of Earth and Space Sciences published a report in *Science* (Cochran *et al.*), which correlated earthquake prevalence with high tides – both water tides and solid land tides. Others have confirmed this correlation: Notably Columbia University's Maya Tolstoy who in 2002 revealed that tidal pressure correlated with deep ocean continental plate earthquakes (Handwerk 2004).

There are also indications that earthquakes and magnetic fields are related. While researchers initially thought of the earth's magnetic fields as rotating above the earth's surface, anisotropic scaling has modeled and measured magnetic fields flowing both vertically and horizontally, even subsurface to the earth's crust. It has been proposed that these changing magnetic fields predispose movement of magma and/or tectonic plates (Moshe 1996).

The amount of the earth's magnetic field ranges from 45,000 to 60,000 nT (nanoTeslas) over the U.S. This huge variance is thought to be created by the existence of "buried magnetic bodies" under the earth's surface. This reality has been confirmed by the fact that magnetic field variances have been found in areas where there is an underground tank or other fixture buried. This especially has been the case for steel underground tanks, which have resulted in variances of thousands of nanoTeslas of magnetic fields. This fact, when combined with anomalies indicated above, points to the probable existence of natural geophysical pockets beneath the earth's surface as discussed above, which might also be construed as active organs or cells.

The active relationships between earthquakes and animals are puzzling yet well known. There have been many verified accounts of animals acting disturbed well in advance of an earthquake. Well before the earthquake can be felt or heard physically – at least to our senses and equipment – animals have evacuated nests, begun running wildly and in general acted erratically. There have been many anecdotal observations of dogs, cats and other animals acting wildly even days before an earthquake. In 1975, the Chinese government evacuated Haicheng based upon the observation of erratic activity by animals. Much of the city was evacuated, and as a result, only minor deaths and injuries occurred from the 7.3-magnitude quake that followed days later.

In 2003, The Quantum Geophysics Laboratory at Osaka University (Yokoi *et al.*) reported that mouse circadian diagrams showed unusual circadian metabolic activity just prior to the 1995 Kobe earthquake. The researchers reported drastic increases in locomotive activity, changes in sleep, and other effects in the mice before the Kobe quake.

As we have mentioned, most animals have an incredible sense of direction and destination. This is witnessed during the incredible migrations of tens of thousands of kilometers by caribou, lobsters, whales, turtles, birds, and so many other organisms. As we described earlier, researchers have found that most of these animals have a sort of magnetic compass within certain cells of the brain and/or spinal cord. Just as a compass needle points north, these animals are able to sense the magnetic fields of the earth using them to create geomagnetic maps of sorts. Birds are apparently able to organize a grid-like mapping of the earth, enabling them to steer back on course around obstacles or weather fronts. Studies of turtles, lobsters, and mole rats have altered magnetic fields, resulting in their reorientation towards the appropriate direction. Mole rats for example, burrow tunnels – sometimes 200 meters long or more – towards the south and place their nests at the end of those burrows. If the magnetic field changes, their burrows will redirect to the southern-most direction of the magnetic field. Loggerhead turtle hatchlings immediately have this sense of direction upon birth. From the beginning of their lives, they are able to sense where to migrate.

While many still insist the universe works through chaos, there is little evidence of this as we observe living organisms traveling a planet under the influence of the sun. We might have assumed living creatures accidentally wander throughout the earth. Yet in reality, our journeys are paced and directed through the geomagnetic fields of the earth. These migratory travels, along with our human physiology, are synchronized with the relative geomagnetic pulses of the sun, moderated by the motion of the solar system, galaxy and universe. Every part of our metabolism, from every cell and enzyme process, is tied to our biomagnetic environment. We have yet to understand precisely how to manipulate biomagnetism from the sun and earth for medical treatment purposes. Perhaps we do not have to nor even want to. Perhaps the best means of utilizing the biomagnetic rhythms from the sun and earth are simply to harmonize out lifestyles with them.

Biomagnetic Strategies

* **Stress:** Both physical and mental stress can easily be linked to a lack of being outside, within nature, where the sun and earth's biomagnetic rhythms flow uninterrupted. The only way we can participate fully with the magnetic flows of nature is to be out there where they influence our bodies directly. This means getting into contact with the earth. This means getting outside into the sun.

* **Indoor lifestyles:** Our modern-day indoor lifestyles have disconnected most of us from nature's biomagnetic influences. As a result, many in the modern world suffer from burdened immune systems, allergies, food sensitivities, a lack of good sleep, lethargy, fibromyalgia, cancer, autoimmune disorder and other degenerative diseases. Our indoor habitats are replete with magnetic influences that disrupt nature's geomagnetic fields.

* **Get grounded:** We can most quickly become connected with the biomagnetic flows of the sun and earth by walking outside barefoot or lying on the ground. We can also sit down on the grass or on a rock when we are outside.

* **Natural fibers:** We can pick wooden or other natural fiber chairs to sit on and walk on indoors. Wood, cotton and stone will resonate with the biomagnetic flows of the earth and sun. By connecting with such materials, our bodies can synchronize with their magnetism. Plastic or other synthetic materials do not resonate with nature's magnetism – one of the central reasons they take so long to decompose.

* **Earth tools:** Utilizing natural materials as tools and utensils is also a good strategy for retaining natural magnetism. We can utilize steel, glass (made of sand) or ceramic plates and bowls for eating. We can use steel silverware. We can utilize wood brushes with natural fibers. We can wear cotton and wool clothing. All of these materials continue to resonate with the geomagnetic flows of the earth and sun – long after they are harvested.

* **Electronics:** Again, distancing our bodies from our electronics, at least periodically, will increase our ability to connect with nature's biomagnetism. We can take off our watches. We can take our cell phones out of our pockets. We can sit back from our computers. We can distance our sleeping environments from the blinking and pulsing of clocks and other electronic appliances.

* **Sensual contact:** We can align with nature's biomagnetic flows by getting into contact with nature with our senses. We can look out the window periodically, smell flowers and dirt, or step outside during our breaks at work. Our senses are biomagnetic in context – they consume geomagnetism.

* **Biomagnetic foods:** Eating unprocessed or raw (or at least minimally processed) foods allows us to literally consume nature's magnetism. Processing interrupts nature's biomagnetism with the electric magnets of motors. It also can exhaust nutrient content by exposing micronutrients to oxygen and light. Whole foods and living foods such as sprouts and yogurt are excellent ways to 'consume' biomagnetism.

* **Get outside:** Once outside, we can reasonably expose our bodies to the sunshine and the other geomagnetic fields coming from space. We can listen to the wind, the birds, and the sound of moving water. We can watch the sunrises, the sunsets, the moonrises, and the nighttime sky's many distant geomagnetic suns.

Chapter Three

Waves of Light

One of the more obvious and overlooked benefits of the sun is light. But what is light? Do we really understand what light is and how the body processes it?

In the seventeenth century, Dutch Christiaan Huygens proposed that light was a wave. A peer of Sir Isaac Newton, Huygens is said to have arrived at this notion by observing wave fronts as they expanded outward and interfered with other wave fronts among the waters of a nearby canal. His observation of wave fronts expanding into their own wavelets seemed to Huygens to correlate nicely with how light might travel.

Sir Newton observed in his research that light was composed not of one simple white ray, but of a spectrum of colors. He demonstrated this by observing light refracting through a prism. Sir Newton also espoused in his 1704 classic *Opticks* that physical objects do not in themselves contain color. Rather, he suggested, color was made of "corpuscles." Some objects absorbed them while other objects reflected them. Those reflected colors, he supposed, created the illusion of that object's color. Sir Newton and Hyugen's works were either largely ignored or refuted vigorously by the mainstream scientific establishment of the time. In Sir Newton's case, though the spectrum was quite visible to the naked eye, criticisms were raised about his research methods and various suppositions.

The light-wave concept was further advanced by Dr. Thomas Young in the late eighteenth century – a century after Huygen's work. Dr. Young observed that if light rays were passed through a slot within a barrier, they would expand outward from the slot. If the same light were shone through two slots in the barrier, the resulting light ray expansions would create both light areas and dark areas on the other side of the barrier – a *diffraction* of light waves. Dr. Young observed that the light rays acted just as water waves might under the circumstances. Two different types of interference patterns emerged as the light shone through the two slots. In some areas, the light waves interacted negatively and dark areas were formed. In other areas, the light waves interacted in such a way that brighter areas resulted.

A few decades later, using calculations based upon earlier discoveries by Faraday and Oersted on the relationship between electric currents and magnetic fields, nineteenth century scientist James Maxwell created a formula implying light not only travels in waves, but also consists of dual electromagnetic waveforms. Using the velocity of light as a measurement basis, his new formula fit the observations of light waves as they exhibited the alternating duality of a wave oscillation. Maxwell and his peers proposed that light's pulsing dual waveform comprised of both electronic and magnetic components, moving perpendicular to each other.

Albert Einstein promoted the concept of light traveling in units with wave-like properties in 1905 with his Nobel Prize-winning paper, *Corpuscular Theory of Light*. Later these same "corpuscular units" espoused by both Newton and Einstein became referred to as *photons* or even *quanta*. Dr. Einstein proposed these photon units carried their energy potential until they encountered atoms within the atmosphere (as he thought space was a vacuum). This encounter would either raise electron orbit energy levels or knock electrons out of atoms' orbits. Either way, the theoretical photon – racing at a theoretically consistent speed – would alter the atom's energy levels following such a collision. Einstein further proposed that photons were of a nature consistent with electron theory of the day: These photons were assumed as being both waves and particles simultaneously. This later became known as the famous *wave-particle theory of light*.

Dr. Einstein's assumption of a consistent speed of light – one of the fundamental assumptions of the quantum view – has hit a snag, however. For over a century physicists have assumed Einstein's proposal that light travels unchanged at close to 300,000,000 meters per second or about 186,000 miles per second. This speed is supposed to be regardless of the frame of reference or location of observation. Collaborative research led by Texas A&M University physics professor Dr. Dimitri Nanopoulos, Dr. Nikolaos Mavromatos of King's College in London, and Dr. John Ellis of the European Center for Particle Physics in Geneva confirmed in 2001 additional influences that alter the speed of light. Their calculations showed that the speed of light actually varies to frequency. Furthermore, in 1999 University of Toronto professor Dr. John Moffat showed evidence that the speed of light has slowed down over time.

Light has been shown to bend via magnetic/gravitational influences as well. Light reflecting from the planet mercury has been seen bending around the sun during a solar eclipse, for example.

Different substances refract and diffract light differently. This is because light will travel with different speeds and vectors through different mediums. As such, each medium has a unique *refractive index*. This relates directly to the substance's molecular makeup. For example, a diamond will refract light differently than a piece of glass might. Water refracts light differently than does air.

Sending light through various substances and then through diffraction gratings based on the principles of Dr. Young have became one of the standard techniques to determine chemical composition or compound purity. A molecule's ability to interfere with the path of light or other radiation as it passes through renders a means for identification. Because light interacts with each atom and molecular structure in a distinct manner, it enables us to quantify this characteristic. This is performed using a *refractometer*.

Visible light waves, for example, have particular polarity, depending upon their source, media and history. Light with different polarity can be *polarized* if its electronic waves and magnetic waves are standardized so that they are consistently at the same angle with the direction of the light. This can be accomplished by refracting the light at specific angles, or simply by viewing the light through a filtering mechanism that screens out waves having different polarity. These methods became the basis for the Polaroid camera and polarized sunglasses, which both screen out unpolarized light waves.

This is not a new concept to nature, however. Various animals and insects see with dramatic polarization. Examples include bees, octopus, and squid, among others. Humans can learn to distinguish light of different polarity with a little training. Because we can see light of particular polarity, our eyes can also conduct some polarization filtration with practice.

Even with all our technology and discovery, our understanding of light is still unfolding. While we might assume our observation of light forms the standard, we may well be missing dramatic pieces of the puzzle, just as Sir Newton missed purple on his color chart.

The Solar Waveplex

The sun produces several types of radiation. They are categorized as visible light rays (from 400 to 700 nm wavelength), infrared radiation (from 750 nm to 1 mm), ultraviolet rays (280 to 400 nm), x-rays (about 10 x -5 nm), gamma rays (10 x -11 to 10 x -14 nm), cosmic rays (10 to 12 cm) and microwaves (1 mm to 30 cm). The earth's atmosphere and the sun's biomagnetic field blocks a good amount of the x-rays, cosmic rays and gamma rays and a significant part of the ultraviolet rays – depending upon the levels of ozone. This allows a good portion of the sun's visible and infrared radiation to hit the surface. In all it is estimated that the atmosphere blocks about 40% of the sun's total radiation.

While many of the rays of the sun can cause damage to the body with over-exposure, ultraviolet radiation has probably received the most attention over recent decades. Ultraviolet-C rays are significantly blocked by the atmosphere. UV-B and UV-A will make it through, however. Between UV-B and UV-A, UV-A rays are more prominent, depending again upon the ozone layer. In most areas, UV-A rays make up over 98% of the ultraviolet radiation that breaks through the atmosphere. The majority of the remainder is UV-B radiation – known best for causing suntans and sunburns.

About half of the heating of the earth's surface is thought to be caused by infrared radiation from the sun. The rest is caused by visible wavelengths of light from the sun being absorbed and radiated to the surface in longer wavelengths. We would propose that these guesstimates do not include the thermal heat generated by the earth itself, which is difficult to measure.

While we can easily separate the colors of the visible radiation into reds, yellows, blues and violets, there are many more colors we cannot see in between and around these wavelengths. Each different waveform stimulates specific sensors in our retinal cells and optic nerves, within a limited range. Different organisms see the sun's light differently as well. For example, bees see ultraviolet light, which assists them in seeing flower pollen.

Artificial Light

In contrast, a typical incandescent light bulb will emit visible light by heating a filament inside a bulb of ionized gas. The filament is usually made of tungsten in an atmosphere of halogens such as nitrogen, krypton, or argon. The incandescent bulb will typically produce three- or four-colored visible light, together with near-infrared waveforms, which create the mild heat typical of a light bulb. Though the bulb will produce visible light, there are various wavelengths missing when comparing to the visible light from the sun. An incandescent bulb typically discharges visible light in the red, green, blue, and violet waveforms. The sun on the other hand, will emit these along with various others, including yellow, purple, turquoise, and so on. For this reason, visible light from the sun allows us to see more colors with better crispness. As these additional waveforms are reflected or absorbed by the objects around us, our eyes see the result.

In addition to these other bands of color waveforms within the visible spectrum, sunlight also emits a full (near and far) ultraviolet and infrared spectrum, along with the other waveforms as mentioned above – many of which are partially filtered as they pass through the atmosphere.

We have had little success trying to duplicate the sun's waveform complex. *"Full spectrum lighting"* is still a far cry from sunlight. Currently there is no real standard for what is called "full-spectrum lighting," so its reference is often misused. There is a quantifying standardization called the *General Color Rendering Index* (or CIE). This gauges the intensity of the color temperature. While red and infrared waveforms are "hot," blue and violet waveforms are considered "cool." A CIE rating that approaches 100 is considered cooler, in that it covers not only some of the ultraviolet waveforms, but also emits at least a range of the main colors such as red, blue, green, and violet.

Tanning bed lighting typically provides primarily ultraviolet radiation. Many tanning lights emit about 95% ultraviolet-A and 5% ultraviolet-B in order to produce the tanning (and burning) equivalent of the sun. Indoor "full spectrum" lights will usually provide some ultraviolet waveforms as well, usually near-ultraviolet, which covers part of ultraviolet-A as well as a decent part of the visual spectrum. Many of the newer "full-spectrum" lamps provide cooler CIE numbers, reflecting a good dose of the blue and green spectrum as well.

Research performed by Rosenthal and Blehar (1989) concluded that lighting with blue and green wavelengths has therapeutic value for *seasonal affective disorder* (SAD). There have also been a number of inconclusive studies on therapeutic "full-spectrum" light. In one review by McColl and Veitch in 2001, research from 1941 through 1999 concluded that "full-spectrum lighting" research has for the most part, not shown any positive effects on either behavior or health – inclusive of hormonal and neural effects. Most researchers have also concluded that there is only marginal vitamin D production from "full-spectrum" lighting. Vitamin D deficiency is one of the more prevalent issues in light-deficiency disorders.

Recent research has confirmed that our bodies also produce light. Dr. Fritz-Albert Popp's work with biophotons over the past few decades has illustrated this effect. Russian researchers V.P. Kaznachejew and L.P Michailowa conducted tests to quantify the transmission and reception of these ultra-weak waveforms. Their conclusions showed that cells and organs produced and received these emissions, and illustrated that information was exchanged between biophotons and other radiation (Schumacher 2005).

Light Spectrography

The electromagnetic nature of light became difficult to argue with after the development of the *crystal field theory* of the 1930s. When light travels through a substance, a portion will be absorbed by the atoms and a portion will be reflected back – depending upon the substance. A ruby looks red because the chromium in the ruby absorbs some of the blue-green wavelengths (around 490 nanometers) while reflecting back a greater amount of red wavelengths (around 650 nanometers). As these 650 nm wavelengths strike the retina, we perceive the color red. This technology is basically the same process of spectroscopy used today by chemists to determine the atomic makeup of a particular molecule or substance. Because atomic particles making up molecules interact distinctively with light, the molecular configuration of a substance can simply be identified by the wavelengths absorbed, reflected, and/or diffracted.

X-ray crystallography and absorption spectroscopy are now two of the most used processes for atomic and molecular identification. Crystallography utilizes the interaction between radiation and substance-matter. X-rays are shot into a crystallized version of a particular substance glued onto the glass of a diffractometer tube. The x-rays react with atoms within the molecular substance and the waveforms of these diffracted rays are recorded onto film or otherwise charted. These diffraction recordings are measured for amplitude and waveform to yield the theoretical atomic structure. Because x-rays are short-wavelength electromagnetic waves, they interact with the electromagnetic waves within the electron clouds. As these interactions occur, they are absorbed or diffracted in a variety of different angles. These angles can be plotted out onto photographic film or computer imagery to display the shape and probable location of the electron clouds.

The resulting crystallographs can indicate any number of angles of wave diffraction. Using diffraction measurements and a formula created by William Bragg and his son in 1913, these plotted angles measure the level of constructive or destructive interference between the x-rays and the sub-atomic particles of the substance. Constructive interference creates a resulting larger wave while destructive interference creates a smaller wave. The type of interference is often a factor of the extent the waves are in-phase or out-of-phase with each other. This in turn relates to polarity, which indicates the possible orientation of the electron cloud.

The interesting thing about spectroscopy is that it is virtually no different from the process our eyes undertake every moment as we look around us. The eyes do not actually see matter. What they see are light rays interacting with and reflecting molecular electromagnetic bonds. It might be compared to looking into a mirror. When we look into a mirror, we are not seeing our actual face. Rather, we are seeing a reflection of our face onto the surface of the mirror.

Solar Waves

When most of us think about waves, we think of the ocean. We think of waves pounding onto the beach. Stirred up by the forces of wind and weather, large waves will march onto the reefs and beaches, standing up with ferocious crests. What we may not realize is that the sun is also pulsing in waves. As we have discussed, the sun pulses electromagnetic waves of different frequencies. The sun also pulses periodic solar storms, each with geomagnetic influence.

Indeed, the sun and the solar system are also moving rhythmically as they circle the Milky Way galaxy in elliptical fashion. Each of these periods form wave shapes, seen when relative positions are graphed against X and Y coordinates.

So what exactly is a wave then?

A wave is a repeating *oscillation:* A translation of information or motion through a particular medium. Waves can travel through solids, fluids, gases, thermals, or electromagnetics. Waves are not restricted to a particular medium, either. Most waves will move through one medium and as that medium connects with another medium, will continue within the next medium. A sound, for example may vibrate a drum skin first. Where the drum skin interacts with air, it oscillates air molecules, creating pressure waves that move information through the air. These pressure waves eventually vibrate the ear's tympanic membrane. The information contained in the waveform is translated to the malleus, incus and stapes of the middle ear. After vibrating through to the round window, the oscillation is translated through the cochlea into nerve pulse oscillations.

Light waves act very similarly, but using electromagnetic waves rather than pressure waves. When sunlight transitions from space to the atmosphere, it is refracted by atmosphere molecules. This refraction alters the waveforms to create light and color. In the same way that the drum translates its oscillations from the drum skin to air pressure waves, light translates its electromagnetic waveforms between the medium of space and the atmosphere. This splinters the electromagnetic waves into visible light and colors.

Every movement in nature has a signature rhythm: The earth oscillates uniquely with seismic waves – some causing damage but most hardly noticeable. We each walk with a signature pace as our feet meet the ground. Our vocal cords oscillate with a pace and timing to form our unique voice. Our heart valves oscillate with our unique circulation requirements. Our lungs oscillate as we breathe in and out – unique to our lung size and cells' needs for oxygen. Even seemingly solid structures like rocks oscillate – depending upon their position, size, shape, and composition. A cliff by the seashore will oscillate with each pounding wave. A building in a windy city will oscillate with the movement of the wind through the streets. Each building will oscillate uniquely, based upon its architecture.

All of these movements – and all movements in nature for that matter – provide recurring oscillations that can be charted in waveform structure. Moreover, the various events within nature come complete with recurring cycles. While many cycles obviously repeat during our range of observation, many cycles have only recently become evident, indicating that many of nature's cycles are beyond our current observation range.

Natural oscillations balance between a particular pivot point and an axis. The axis is a frame of reference between two media or quanta. An axis showing quantification may illustrate time in reference to height, time versus temperature, time versus activity or time versus other quantifying points of reference. Waves will also conduct between media. The ocean wave is created by the transferring of waveforms between the atmosphere and water. The water's surface tension gives rise to the ocean wave as it refracts the pressure of wind from a storm system. The storm system's waveform will eventually conduct through the ocean to the rocks and beach.

Nature's waves are relational to the rhythms of planets and galaxies. These rhythms translate to electromagnetic energy and kinetic energy, which translate to the elements of speed, distance, and mass. Momentum, inertia, gravity, and other natural phenomena are thus examples of the cyclical activities that directly relate with nature's wave rhythms. Every rhythm in nature is interconnected with other rhythms. Like a house built with interconnected beams of framing, the universe's rhythms are all interconnected with a design of pacing within the element of time.

The most prevalent waveform found in nature is the sinusoidal wave. The sinusoidal wave is the manifestation of circular motion related to time. Thus, the sine wave repeats through nature's processes defined by time. For example, the rotating positions of the hands of a clock translate to a sinusoidal wave should the angles of the hand positions be charted on one axis with the time on the other axis. Light moves with this sinusoidal motion.

Sinusoidal waveforms are also the predominant structures for sound, electromagnetic waves and ocean waves. Late eighteenth and early nineteenth century French physicist Jean Fourier found that just about every motion could be broken down into sinusoidal components. This phenomenon has become known as the *Fourier series*.

The cycle of a sine wave, moving from midline to a peak, then back to midline then to a trough and back to the midline completes a full cycle. If we divide the wave into angles, the beginning is consistent with 0 degrees; the first peak is consistent with 45 degrees, the midline with 90 degrees and the trough with 270 degrees. This creates a circle, and each revolution around the circle is a complete sine wave cycle.

Other wave types occurring in nature might not be strictly sine waves, yet they are often sinusoidal in essence. The cosine wave, for example, is sinusoidal because it has the same basic shape, but is simply *phase-shifted* from the sine. Other waves such as square waves or irregular sound waves can usually be connected to sinusoidal origin when their motion is broken down into composites.

We see so many circular activities within nature. We see the earth recycling molecular components. We see the recycling of water from earth to sea to clouds and back to earth. We see planetary bodies moving in cyclic fashion, repeating positions in periodic fashion. We see the seasons moving in cyclic repetition. We see organisms living cycles of repetitive physical activity.

While not every cycle in nature is precisely circular – the orbits of planets or electron energy shells for example – they are nonetheless revolving within a cyclic fashion. Linked cycles often contain various alterations as they adapt to the other cyclic components. This modulation can be described as adaptation – a harmonic process observed among both matter and life.

This all should remind us of the notion of the circle of life, which has been repeatedly observed throughout nature in so many respects that it is generally assumed without fanfare. Circles recur in human and animal activity, social order, customs, and individual circumstances. We cycle emotionally and psychologically. The tribal circle is common among many ancient cultures – and for good reason. In modern society, we have circular conferences, round-table meetings, and cyclical ceremonies. The potter's wheel, the grinding wheel, and the circular clock are all examples of circular symbols in our attempt to synchronize with nature. Just about every form of communication and transportation is somehow connected to circular motion. For this reason, it is no accident that the wheel provides our primary means for transportation. The motion of walking is also circular/sinusoidal, as the legs rise and fall forward, rotating the various joints. And the sun, of course, is a circular disc.

In nature, we observe two basic types of waves: Mechanical and electromagnetic. A mechanical wave moves through a particular medium: sound pressure waves as they move through air, for example. Mechanical waves can move over the surface of a medium. Ocean waves and certain earthquake (seismic) waves are examples of mechanical surface waves. Another type of mechanical wave is the tortional wave: This mechanical wave twists through a spiral or helix.

The electromagnetic wave is seemingly different because it theoretically does not move through a medium of any composition. Einstein physics assumes space is a vacuum and the sun's electromagnetic waves move through this vacuum. A heady debate regarding the content of the medium of space took place during the late nineteenth and early twentieth centuries. Dr. Einstein's proposal that space is a vacuum was followed with theories of special relativity. According to the theory, time and space in this vacuum of space are collapsed: Instead of time and distance being separate, they become a singular element of space-time. However, now that we know the speed of light is not constant, the notion of a wave being able to travel through a totally collapsed vacuum would be inconsistent with the mechanics of time.

Nature displays two basic waveform structures: transverse and longitudinal. Visible spectrum, radiowaves, microwaves, radar, infrared and x-rays are all transverse waveforms. As these waves move, there is a disruption moving at right angles to the vector of the wave. For example, should the wave move along a longitudinal x-axis, its disruption field would move in the perpendicular y-z axes. This might be compared to watching a duck floating on a lake strewn with tiny waves. The duck bobs up and down as the waves pass under the duck's body. The bobbing would be analogous to the magnetic field vectors of the sun's electromagnetic waves.

The other waveform is longitudinal. Here pressure gradients form regular alternating zones of compression and rarefaction. During the compression phase, the medium is pressed together, and during the rarefaction, the medium is expanded outward. This might be illustrated by the alternating expansion and compression of a spring. Instead of the wave disturbing the medium upward and downward as in the case of a transverse wave, the medium is disturbed in a back and forth fashion in the direction of the wave. Examples of longitudinal waves are seismic waves and sound waves. In the case of sound waves, air molecules compress and rarefy in the direction of the sound projection.

These two types of waves coherently combine in nature. An ocean wave is a good example of a combination of transverse and longitudinal waveforms. Water may be disturbed up and down as it transmits an ocean wave, and it may convey alternating compressions and rarefaction as it progresses tidal currents.

Waves are typically referred to as radiation when the waveform can translate its energy information from one type of medium to another. In this respect, seismic waves and ocean waves can be considered radiating as they translate their energy onto the sand in the case of ocean waves, or through buildings in the case of seismic waves. The classic type of radiation comes from electromagnetic waves such as x-rays or ultraviolet rays, which can travel through skin or other molecular mediums after transversing space.

Waves are typically measured by their wave height from trough to crest (amplitude), rate of speed through time (frequency) and the distance from one repeating peak to another (wavelength). Waves also may have specific wave shapes such as sinusoidal, square, or otherwise.

The frequency of a wave is typically measured by how many wave cycles (one complete revolution of the wave) pass a particular point within a period of time. Therefore, waves are often measured in CPS, or cycles per second. The *hertz* is named after nineteenth century German physicist Dr. Heinrich Hertz, who is said to have discovered radio frequency electromagnetic waves. Note that hertz and cps are identical: Both the number of complete waves passing a given point every second. Other frequency measurements used include machinery's RPM (revolutions per second), special radiation's RAD/S (radians per second), and the heart's BPM (beats per minute).

Wavelength is frequently measured in meters, centimeters, or nanometers to comply with international standards. Each radiation type is classified by its wavelength. A wave's wavelength has an inverse relationship to its frequency. This is because a shorter wave's length will travel faster through a particular point than a longer length will. Note also that speed is the rate measured from one point to another, while frequency is the rate of one full repetition to another past a particular point. Therefore, a wave's wavelength can be determined by dividing its speed by its frequency. Of course, a wave's speed can also be divided by its wavelength to obtain the frequency.

Despite popular science literature's penchant for naming only one aspect of a particular wave (often either wavelength or frequency), we must consider the various other specifications of a particular wave to have a useful understanding of it. When we describe a sinusoidal waveform, however, we can state either its frequency or wavelength, since the two will be inversely related. Otherwise, the wave's amplitude is an important consideration, as this relates to the height of the wave from peak to trough. Among sinusoidal waves, larger amplitude will accompany a larger wavelength. We also might consider the specific phase of a wave, its medium of travel, and again its wave shape. These together will help us arrive at a more precise set of specifications to more accurately describe the nature of a particular wave. While one or more of these specifications might be used to describe a particular wave in popular media, in reality all should be considered. Here we refer to a unique combination of these specifications with the term *waveform*.

Waves travel with some form of repetition or periodicity. The very definition of a wave describes a repeating motion of some type. This repetition, occurring with a particular pace and particular time reference, together forms a rhythm. All around us, we see wave rhythms. Can waves be chaotic? To the contrary, it is their very consistent, non-chaotic rhythm that allows us to interpret light, color, sound, or warmth with precision. All of these waveforms connect with the senses because they have consistent and congruent oscillations. In sensing the world around us, we do not perceive each wave individually. Rather, we perceive the information contained in multiple, interactive waves.

When a waveform collides or *interferes* with another waveform, the result is often a more complex form of information: A combination of the two. As waveforms collide throughout our universe, they comprehensively present a myriad of complex information conductance. This information is only available to us to the extent we can sense and interpret those interference patterns, however.

We can thus surmise that nature is composed of various combinations and interactions of these two types of waves (longitudinal and transverse) with various waveforms. The classic waveforms vibrating through space and radiating through physical molecules may be fairly easy for us to isolate, chart and measure. Within nature however, waves collide and interfere with each other to create interference patterns we cannot always interpret. Colliding waves interfere with each other's continuing motion in some way, forming a multitude of complexity.

The more precise reason why not all waves are obviously sinusoidal is that nature is complicated by these different types of interactions between different types of waveforms. When dissimilar waveforms collide, there is a resulting disturbance or interference pattern. Depending upon the characteristics of the two colliding waveforms, this interference could result in a larger, complex waveform – or constructive interference pattern. Alternatively, should the waveforms contrast each other; their meeting could cause a resultant reduction of waveforms – a destructive interference pattern. The ability of two waves to interact to form a greater waveform lies within their similarity of wave phase. If one wave is cycling in positive territory while the other is cycling in negative territory as the two collide, they will most likely destructively interfere in each other, canceling some or all of their effects. However, if the two waves move in the same phase – where both cycle with the same points on the curve – then they will most likely constructively interfere with each other.

As a result, interference between waves can be in phase or they can be out of phase. In phase waveforms will often meet with superposition to form larger, more complex waveforms. Out of phase waveforms will often conflict, reducing, and canceling part of their effective rhythms in one or many ways. This canceling or reduction of interfering waves is not necessarily bad, however. Destructive interference can also communicate various types of information.

The degree that two or more waves will interfere with each other – either constructively or destructively – is their coherence. In other words, if two waves are coherent, they will greatly affect each other, creating either a greater resulting pattern or a canceling and reducing pattern between them. Waves that are too different to create any significant interference are said to be incoherent. This term usage is very similar to how we describe comprehension in language. Coherent sounds generally mean the sounds are better understood by the listener. Whether the communication is interpreted by the listener positively or negatively, the clarity of the communication is indicative of its coherence. This is analogous to coherence in wave mechanics. Coherent waves interfere either constructively or destructively as they interact.

Resonance occurs when individual waves are expanded to a balanced state – one where the amplitude and period is the largest for that waveform system. Thus, resonating waves typically occur when waves come together in constructive interference. This results in a maximization of their respective wave periods and amplitudes. This is illustrated when two tuned instruments play the same note or song together. Their strings will resonate together, creating a convergence with greater amplitude, which will typically (depending of course upon the surrounding environment) result in a louder, clearer sound. We also see (or hear) this when we create the familiar whistling sound accomplished by blowing into a bottle spout: To get the loudest sound, we must blow with a certain angle and airspeed – positioning our lips with the shape of the bottle. Once we find the right positioning, angle and speed, we have established a resonance.

As waves move from one media to the next, they will partially reflect or refract. Reflected waves will bounce off the new medium, while refracted waves will move through a new medium with a different vector and speed, depending upon the density and molecular makeup of the medium. The result may be diffraction – a break up of the vector direction of the rays. The ability of a particular medium to provoke these changes is referred to as its index of refraction. Some mediums will reflect certain waveforms while refracting others. In many cases, the medium will reflect some and refract some of the waves. Most mediums will also absorb certain types of waveforms, as we will discuss further. The type of waveforms reflected and absorbed will usually determine the medium's perceived color and clarity.

The sun's waves will be both refracted and reflected by the atmosphere. Some of the waves, such as cosmic rays and gamma waves, and many UV-B rays, will be reflected or absorbed by the molecules of the earth's outer atmosphere. This effectively blocks their entry into our inner atmosphere. Other sun rays will enter the atmosphere and be refracted. Still others will be diffracted. Rainbows are good examples of sun rays that have been refracted by water molecules within the earth's atmosphere.

Diffraction occurs when the sun's rays interfere with or otherwise accommodate a group of static waveforms. This interference accommodation results in a bending and disbursement of the rays of light, somewhat similar to refraction. The difference is that diffraction results in a completely different waveform structure and visual image. For example, the diffraction of the sun's rays by the moon will create a halo or aura around the moon. Diffraction is also the principle that modern-day holographic pictures work.

Water illustrates the refraction, reflection and diffraction of the sun's rays quite well. Part of the sun's UV-A, UV-B and visible light rays will refract or bounce off the water, while the rest enters the water. For this reason, sunning next to water will increase UV-B exposure. Sunbathing next to water will often burn the skin because of this increased intensity of UV-B (from both the sun and water reflection). Because UV refracts and diffracts through water, it is also possible to pick up a tan or even burn within shallow water. As one goes deeper, however, the UV rays are diffracted from the water's own mechanical wave motion. This interference disperses the UV rays within a few feet of water to the point where their tanning or burning capacity is minimized.

In deeper water, transverse and longitudinal wave motions combine to form monochromatic linear plane waves. This is a type of wave called an inertial wave. Inertial waves are typically moving within rotating fluid mediums. Inertial waves are common in not only the ocean and lakes, but also within the atmosphere and presumably within the earth's core. The various currents and winds within the atmosphere all travel in varying length inertial waves. These inertial waves also create various diffractions from the sun's rays as they travel towards the earth's surface. This creates a variety of colors in the sky, including the sky's blueness.

Diffraction also creates the wonderful orange, purple and even red skies we adore during sunsets and sunrises. During these times, particles that are normally absent due to the heat of the day or the angle of the sun fall in the line of sight of the sun's rays. The sun's rays then diffract and scatter around these particles, forming the multitude of colors of sunsets and sunrises.

A simple harmonic is a recurring wave (usually sinusoidal) that repeats its own rhythmic frequency. When different waveforms converge and their frequencies are aligned – they are multiples or integers of each other – their waveform combination becomes harmonized: There is a mathematical integral multiple between them. In other words, harmony is based upon waveforms having a multiple of the same fundamental base. For example, waveforms with frequencies at multiples of a particular waveform will harmonize.

As forward-moving waves interact with returning waves, both waves will become compressed and dilated. This is known as the *Doppler effect* – named after nineteenth century Austrian physicist Johann Christian Doppler. If the incoming waves have the same waveform, frequency, and amplitude, this will create a standing wave. If they do not, either the incoming or the outgoing wave will divert the waves it meets, and distort those waves in one respect or another.

Standing waveforms will typically have the same frequency, wavelength, amplitude, and shape as they oscillate. This creates a balance and resonance that gives the perceiver (using retinal perception) the illusion that those standing waves are solid objects.

As suggested by Zhang *et al.* in 1996, and confirmed by multiple physicists over the last decade, multiple electrons within shared orbitals among multiple atoms situated within a close-range matrix are best described as multiple standing waves: These are standing waveforms within minute space. They create some of the strongest forces in nature, as they compile the illusion of physical reality. The convergence of these multiple waveforms standing together in a harmonic resonating pattern for a unique period of time is best described as architecture.

Harmonic synchronized and resonating waveforms create structure and consistent chemical properties among electrons, protons, atoms and molecules. The convergence or interference displacement among bonding orbitals and electromagnetic waves conveys order and mathematical precision. Our world is composed of this orderly nature, and the electromagnetic waveforms from the sun support that order.

This is because the waveforms from the sun resonate coherently with the atomic and molecular 'receptors' within nature. The waves of the sun move through nature with waveform coherence. They resonate coherently with molecules within plants, stimulating photosynthesis and creating color. They resonate with all molecules to produce heat. They resonate coherently with our photoreceptors to create our visions of nature. They resonate with the various receptors of our skin cells to raise our body core temperature and stimulate our pineal gland. Special skin cell receptors receive ultraviolet radiation to produce vitamin D – as we will discuss in depth later.

These receptors in effect echo the rays of the sun throughout our internal and external environments. This resonation with the sun's rays floods these environments just as a tsunami will drench every tree and organism once it connects with the shore.

What this all means is that when we see color among the objects around us, we are actually seeing the sun: The sun's rays are reflecting and diffracting through the molecules of every object. Even among fire or incandescent lights, we are seeing these "fires" in the form of energy and combustion. These waveforms have a particular wavelength, amplitude and frequency that resonate with the photoreceptor neurons (rods and cones) within our retinas. The waveforms corresponding to different colors are absorbed by different receptors. Our visual cortex and mental programming interpret absorption populations as different colors and objects.

As we interpret particular colors among the plants and materials of nature, we are realizing coherence among the waveforms coming from the sun (or indirectly in the form of fire or incandescent lighting). There is coherence between the sun's waveforms and the natural objects we see as color. There is also a direct coherence between the sun's waveforms and the photoreceptors of our eyes.

It is important to remember that while the earth travels in an elliptical-circular path around the sun, the sun is also traveling an elliptical-circular path within a spiraling Milky Way. We might also consider that our preliminary indications of the structure of atoms and molecules also appear to have similar elliptical-circular orbiting pathways. While many consider this coincidence, it is more logically a display of coherence and resonance within the universe. The patterns of motion are coherently resonating through the larger and smaller regions of the universe.

Indeed the sun also appears round to our eyes – despite the fact that solar flares and magnetic fields stream outward to make variable shapes. We should also remember that our eyes are elliptically circular, encouraging the circular appearance of larger, far-away objects. Practically any lens we utilize also encourages circular images. We can compare this to peering up while underwater within a round barrel. Many objects outside and above the barrel will take on a round or circular appearance. This is because the light rays are refracting through the water – bending inward towards our round eyes. We might therefore conclude that the elliptical/circular perception of the sun may at least be contributed by the fact that our eyes, lenses, planet and solar system are all elliptical/circular.

We might compare the limitation of our eyes with how limited an ant's eyes might be relative to ours. For example, an ant would likely see a table lamp as being a large circular orb because of the intensity of light the lamp throws off relative to the rest of the lamp's assembly. The ant would likely not be able to perceive the design qualities of the lamp itself, as those would be beyond the ant's scope. The lamp, therefore, would appear to the ant much as the sun might appear to our eyes – a bright circular orb.

The Spiral Solar System

Spirals are inherent in nature. For example, when we see the rhythmic spiraling growth of leaves or branches in Fibonacci sequence around the trunk of a tree we are presented with an interference of Fibonacci waveforms and the vectors of growth coming from the living plant. This interference creates a spiral or helix pattern of leaves growing upward and/or outward. Should we spread out the spiral orientation of a plant into two dimensions – x and y coordinates – we would find that the branching reflects a sinusoidal wave pattern. Should we look down at the plant from its apex, we would see this spiraling or helical effect, depending upon the size and nature of the plant. Looking at a younger plant – where we could see the top shoots with respect to the bottom trunk – we might perceive a spiral. Should we look at a larger tree with a large trunk at the bottom with its branches swirling and widening to the top, we might perceive a helix.

These helical and spiraling forms provide the basic structures for life within the physical world. We see these structures present from the smallest elements of life to the largest elements, from the double helixed DNA molecule to the spiraling galaxies of the universe. We see the spiral within all types of anatomical shapes. The nautilus shell is most famous, but just about every shell formation also reflects this spiraling nature. The swirling of tornadoes, hurricanes, and weather systems mirror this spiral as well. Our senses are also tied to rotational spheres and spirals. Our cochlear hearing system utilizes a spiral to convert air pressure waves to neuron impulses. Our eyes are circular, spiraling through the pupils to the retina, bending light with filtration before they hit the retinal cells. When we consider the twisting and bending path of light through our visual senses, we ultimately arrive at the trigonometric sinusoidal and spiral. Other displays of nature's spiraling energies include the magnetic fields of the earth; animal displays of spiraling structures such as claws, teeth, horns, irises, ear pinea, and fingerprints.

In fact, there is good reason to believe that the sun's electromagnetic rays are spirals rather than waves. While a pulsed wave would be perceived looking at a side view of a moving wave, an x-y-z chart would show another perspective. Our light models all indicate that the magnetic fields are moving outward *three-dimensionally*. This means that if we were to look directly at the radiation from the sun – modeled of course – we would see them swirling towards us, quite similar to looking through a tube or funnel – or perhaps even a tornado from the bottom.

Just as the sinusoid wave is derived from the circle, the classic spiral may be derived from the sphere. Beginning at any one of a sphere's apexes or poles, a spiral is formed if we move around the curvature of the sphere towards the opposite poles. Hence, this most basic type of spiral is known as the spherical spiral. The spherical spiral is also known as the arithmetic or Archimedean spiral, named after the third century B.C.E. Greek mathematician Archivedes of Syracuse. In this spiral, the distance between each layer (or spiral arm) is held equidistant. This creates an angular moment that is consistent throughout.

There are various other types of spirals in nature. The Fibonacci sequence is often displayed within either helical or spiral forms. Fibonacci spirals are close relatives to the logarithm spiral. Fermat's spiral – named after sixteenth century Frenchman Pierre de Fermat – is related to the arithmetic spiral. In 1979, Helmut Vogel proposed variant of Fermat's spiral as a better approximation of nature's Fibonacci spiral. This is the spiral observed within phyllotaxis forms, which include sunflowers, daisies and certain spiraling universes. Around 1638, Rene Descartes revealed the equiangular spiral. This spiral reflects geometrical radii outward as polar angles increase. The relationship Descartes discussed ($S=AR$, which Evangelista Torricelli also developed independently during that era) has also been called the geometrical spiral. Edmond Halley's seventeenth and eighteenth century work revealed the proportional spiral. Jacob Bernoulli developed its logarithmic basis, revealing the logarithmic spiral shortly thereafter. Bernoulli gave it the namesake of *spira mirabilis,* meaning "wonderful spiral." It is said Bernoulli's fascination of the spiral led to his request it be engraved on his tombstone. We note also Bernoulli's famous work with water pressure, and of course the water funnel – or water spout.

As pointed out by Giuseppe Bertin and C.C. Lin in their 1996 book *Spiral Structure in the Galaxies*, the spiraling galaxies may well be generated through a combination of density waves that rotate in a slower rhythm than the rest of the galaxy's various stars, planets and gases. The *density wave theory*, first proposed in 1964 by C.C. Lin and Frank Shu, explains that the harmonization of the angular paths and the mutual gravitational attraction of the galaxy's components form areas of greater density. This allows the spiral arm formation without a *winding problem.*

Much of nature is arranged in helix or spiral shape. What may not appear to be is most likely should we peer through its cross-section. For example, an ocean wave breaking over a reef may appear to be a half waveform as it is looked at straight on from the beach. However, a cross-sectional view of the same wave reveals its spiral motion: As we watch the water falling from one side of the crest – crashing into the trough from the side, the spiral effect comes into view. The combination of the forward movement of the wave to the beach and the sideways movement of water along the crest creates the surfer's classic spiraling *tube* or *barrel.* To ride the tube or barrel requires the surfer to stay just ahead of the final eclipsing of the water with the trough. Should the surfer lapse into the center point of the spiral, the surfer will most likely be separated from the surfboard and experience the *wipe out.*

The hurricane is a similar example of this effect. Waves from two different pressure and temperature fronts interact to form the classic cyclone effect seen from satellite. The hurricane and weather system spirals are only visible from above. This means for thousands of years, humankind had no direct awareness of this spiraled form. Looking at a hurricane front from the land renders a view of the coming front 'wave' of rain and wind from the storm. While many speculated about weather systems as they experienced the 'eye of a hurricane,' and compared this with that other classic spiraling interaction of waveforms – the tornado – it was only as humans began to take to the air that these beautiful spiraling images unveiled themselves.

D'Arcy Wentworth Thompson's 1917 classic *On Growth and Form,* and Sir T.A. Cook's 1903 *Spirals in Nature and Art* both illustrated the many examples of nature's tremendously precise spiraling waveform elements. Mr. Thompson details how various elements in nature have a tendency to coil, such as hair, tails, elephant trunks and cordiform leaves among others. Other interesting helix and spiral movements include the spiraling burrowing of rodents and the spiral swimming of dolphins and whales.

Let us not forget nature's molecular spirals and helixes. The most famous of which is DNA and RNA – storing and processing the programming of metabolism. The discovery of DNA, ironically, was determined through the use of crystallography, which diffracted x-rays through the molecule's distinct bonding patterns.

In 1973, Dr. Michael Rossmann reported the finding of a protein structure where multiple coiling strands are linked together with two helical structures. The connection between the strands and the helices were found to be alternating, forming an available structure for nucleotide bonding. This structure proved to be an important helical structure: Nicotinamide adenine dinucleotide (NAD) is a critical coenzyme involved in the production of energy and genetic transcriptional processing within every living cell.

We have since found that numerous other biochemical molecular structures are actually helical when we are able to observe their *tertiary* structure. Various polysaccharides, polypeptides, hormones, neurotransmitters and fatty acids produced by the various living species have helical molecular structures. Many electron clouds have also proved to have helical or spiral shape. Certainly, this spiraling micro universe of atoms and molecules would have astounded the generations of thoughtful scientists over the centuries.

At the same time, physicists have been disturbed by the *paradox of the spiral.* This issue was noted by Dr. Einstein, who concluded this in discussion of the related *Faraday disc problem,* as apparently a radial conductance: *"It is known that Maxwell's electrodynamics – as usually understood at the present time – when applied to moving bodies, leads to asymmetries that do not appear to be inherent in the phenomena."* He went on to propose that "asymmetry" arises when the currents are produced without a "seat" of forces. As we have previously discussed, the magnetic field tends to exert a force vector moving perpendicular to that of electrical current. As this happens, angular momentum is inferred from the induction. When the torque of angular momentum arising from the conducting Faraday Disc is considered together coherently interacting currents and fields, the dynamic of the spiral becomes evident (Serra-Valls 2007).

If we overlay nature's spiraling motion within the cyclical structure of the molecular world, a tremendous symphony of alignment becomes apparent. As we observe this mysterious collection of movement and symmetry, we naturally seek to find the basis for the underlying tendency of nature to coherently interact with a twisting wave motion concluding in rhythmic spirals and helixes. Dr. Einstein proposed that we accept that many of the movements of nature are either moving relatively too fast or too slow for us to observe. We can apply this to our understanding of the sun's wavelike, spiraling oscillations. For this reason, we find our research only gives us momentary glimpses of the complex harmonic existing within our solar system.

We can ponder more deeply the reality that a sphere is really a three-dimensional circle. When we measure radiation on oscilloscopes or computerized data, we are essentially measuring a two-dimensional view of a force that likely has a third dimension. Playing out this perspective illustrates that the magnetic field moving away perpendicular to the electronic vector in any electromagnetic wave would create a helical and spiraling arrangement.

Regarding the apparent differences between the spiral and the helix, we point out that when cross-referenced with the axes of time and space, a helix will convert to a spiraled helix. This may require a cross-sectional view to complete the image, however – just as we explained with a beach break wave. If we are looking at the wave fully breaking (say a *"close out"* wave) at once, we see a cylinder from the beach. It is the view from the wave, looking down the length of the wave from the side that brings the spiral into view. In the same way, as time and space accumulates helical motion along one axis or another, we observe that one end of the helix will be more relevant than the other end. This progression may also be perceived as the helical arms expanding outward as the helix approaches us. Even without this relativity of motion towards the perceiver, we can understand this effect.

We can illustrate the effect of time and space in motion by observing a train approaching us. The front of the train as it approaches us is closer and thus appears larger than the rest of the train. Though the train size is consistent through all the cars, our perception at that point of time is of a large locomotive and small caboose. In the same way, would we be able to travel through time within the motion of the spiral, we would arrive at a helix from our perspective, and vice versa in the inverse. Likewise, a person caught in the eye of a hurricane or tornado will not perceive the funneling shape of the storm. The helical or spiral view would only be perceivable from a distance or from above, respectively.

Most consider rhythms to be exclusively a characteristic of music. Certainly, a gathering of interference patterns between harmonious rhythms creates a melodious song. Is this not what the sun is generating? All of the various waveforms of color, temperature, wind, motion, sound, heat and light are radiating through their interference with the sun's spiraling waveforms, forming a symphony of activity on our planet. Our bodies are tuned to resonate with this symphony.

Coherent Radiation

The discovery and utilization of electromagnetic frequency has enabled humans to successfully communicate sounds and images with precision over long distances. Contrary to popular thinking, radiowaves, microwaves, x-rays and others were not invented: They were discovered. The sun produces these forms of radiation. Their discovery simply allowed humans to utilize radiation to communicate over longer distances. Pictures and sounds are converted to electronic pulses and broadcast to distant receivers. Once received, the pulses are converted back to sound or picture images through resistance and transistance using semiconductors and integrated circuits. At first glace these communications may seem incredibly technical. Once we stumbled upon these different forms of natural radiation after tinkering with electricity for a couple of centuries, we were able to utilize and manipulate the sun's technology. We can see this in the various contributions of many scientists who developed these communication systems. Hundreds, even thousands of researchers have tapped into these natural waveforms in one respect or another. In the end, we can thank the ambitions of a few scientist-businessmen for our modern communications technologies.

We should note that the discovery of radiated communications and our ability to use it has not necessarily been the result of our understanding it. The development of radio wave signaling by Gugielmo Marconi and Ferdinand Braun during the late nineteenth and early twentieth centuries led to the 1909 Nobel Prize in Physics for the wireless telegraph. The telegraph was developed over a hundred years earlier through the combined tinkering of Francisco de

Salva, Alessandro Volta, Samuel von Soemmering and Johan Schweigger. These efforts began with simple electrostatics. This further developed into the manipulation of currents and voltage. Heinrich Hertz introduced the existence and detection of electromagnetic radiation in the late 1880s. An Italian physicist and university professor Augusto Righi investigated their optical properties in the years following. He published no less than 200 papers on the subject. While Marconi developed methods of electric wave propagation, it was Righi who improved upon the technology. Righi was able to increase wave stability and reception clarity.

Edouard Branly, utilizing some of the work of Italian physicist Temistocle Calzecchi-Onesti, eventually assembled a crude radio transmitter. This became referred to as the *Branly coherer*. It utilized current resistance to transmit alternating radiowaves across an electrode. It was Englishman Dr. Oliver Lodge who coined the term *coherer*, postulating that the medium through which the radiowaves transmitted was the *aether*. Dr. Lodge is thought to have demonstrated wireless transmission prior to Marconi; and quite possibly Nikola Tesla may have demonstrated the first wireless radio wave communication in 1893.

The key element was added around 1898 by German Ferdinand Braun, however. Braun invented the *cat's whisker-crystal diode rectifier*. This formed the basis for the *crystal radio receiver*, which utilized a natural crystal as a semiconductor. The natural crystal was positioned to receive and conduct radiowaves through contact with a thin bronze wire – the *cat's whisker*.

Eventually a tuner was installed to fix the radio crystal and whisker upon a particular station emitting radiowave pulses. The crystal semiconductor converted these waveforms into electrical pulses, driving a speaker. Marconi, the ultimate businessperson, assembled the various equipment – much of it under patent by the original inventors – and combined them with existing telegraph technology to send and translate real-time communication.

It should be noted that the signaling system on both ends must be grounded to the earth: Nature provides not only the facility for semi-conductance but also the grounding for the electrical pulses to provide the right polarity. Early semiconducting devices were made from crystals of natural minerals such as galena or pyrite. Prior to the cat's whisker crystal radio, other minerals like silicon carbide and vitreous silicon were also used as crude semiconductors. All of these of course preceded the use of elemental silicon for the semi-conduction of integrated circuit and microchip technology.

The ability to broadcast communications riding on the band-widths of nature's radiowaves was an invention of equipment only. The equipment enabled humans to utilize natural radiation as a car-rier for information communication. With various experiments and mechanisms developed through trial and error, inventors and physi-cists have been able to build upon this natural technology. The technology itself is utilized by nature through the transmission of voice, energy, and heat. Moreover, if we examine the timeline of the inventions and some of the theories proposed by Bohr, Einstein, de Broglie, and others, the mechanical ability thoroughly preceded humankind's understanding of radiation technologies. As we have discussed, physicists are still debating many of the basic theories regarding radiation and communications. In other words, we still do not completely understand these natural waveform technologies.

Radiation transmission is really an innate rhythmic process natural to all living beings. Radiation communication can be com-pared to the barking of a dog, or the tapping of Morse code. The sending of the signal is the act of the tapping or barking, and the receiving of the signal is the act of sensing or hearing those rhyth-mic waveforms, followed by a translation of the information communicated. This allows the sender and receiver to have an in-tended communication, filtering out other communications with a *handshaking* protocol. As long as each party agrees on how the rhythm is to be converted, communication can be extensive and personal.

A television camera converts visual data into a series of digital pulses. Those pulses are converted through electricity into broad-cast radiowaves. A television set is the receiver and converter of those radiowaves, translating the pulses back into digital mode. As long as the television receiver is set up with the same conversion coding (or handshaking) used in the camera to broadcast signal conversion, it can convert the pulses into the right images.

If we were to analyze voice or even Morse code on a two-dimensional oscilloscope, we will see the same thing we see when we look at an electronic broadcast transmission: A series of wave-forms. As a signal is converted from electronic broadcast pulses to voice and pictures, the information contained in the waveforms are converted from one carrier system (radiowaves) to another (digital integrated circuitry). During this conversion, the information is conserved as the waveform is translated from radio wave to elec-tronic pulse. It is these pulses that are eventually converted to projected pictures and sound waves. This is the transmission of information through radiation. The information is the energy being transmitted and the waveform media are its carriers.

Photosynthesis is the natural version of waveform radiation transmission and conversion. Sunlight wave pulses are converted by photosynthesis into the nutritional building blocks and energy needed by the plant utilizing biomolecular reactions to convert the sun's radiation. Biomolecular reactions convert one molecule to another while releasing and/or absorbing energy. Each living organ-ism has this capability of converting radiation through biomolecular reaction. The conversion of the sun's radiation is the fundamental metabolic and informational waveform process of all organisms.

All organisms receive, convert and transmit informational wave-forms of variety of types. Dolphins and many whales, for example, can not only code and transmit through sound, but they can utilize informational waveform signals to echo-locate – obtaining three-dimensional pictures of surrounding objects or creatures. This sense is typically referred to as sonar, which stands for SOund Navigation And Ranging. Sonar allows these intelligent creatures the ability to analyze an object's shape, movement, and location from very long distances. While research has long confirmed that dolphins and whales use sonar, it now appears they may have the ability to sense the feelings and emotions of other animals during these complex sound wave transmissions.

Even ants communicate through a complex coding system of touching each other's antennae. Other animals can broadcast re-ports and emotions over many miles. They can announce their proprietary territories along with their state of affairs with complex sounds. When a dog's domain is faced with a threatening situation, for example, he can broadcast that situation out to other dogs in that area. Those dogs can in turn broadcast the information to other regions if necessary. Theoretically, remote dog populations can almost instantly know a single dangerous situation through a relay of sound transmission.

This illustrates how broadcasting and reception technologies are simply an extension of natural processes. Just as the ears are equipped with a converting mechanism in the form of the bones of the ear and the cochlear hair that translate sound frequencies into nervous impulses, our gigantic radio telescopes receive transmissions from deep space and attempt to convert this into useful data. The same operation is taking place, except that the telescope technology has not been able to translate much meaning from the many space signals. While both are simply conversion instruments, the translation technology of telescope computers is no match for the complex technologies of our natural sense mechanisms.

Different sense organs translate light, sound and tactile waveforms. These waveforms allow us to receive information from a variety of energy sources. These information waveforms provide the basic platform for structure within our universe. The information carried through waveforms of various types connects everything together with resonation and coherence – aligning molecular waveforms into sequential progression. This provides an environment designed for learning.

The ability to broadcast intended information through waveform radiation is well established. We can communicate intention within sound waves. We can broadcast intention within radiowaves. We can deliver healing intentions or destructive intentions within lasers, x-rays and atomic energy. Just as the waves of the ocean can carry a surfer or a boat, we can ride these waveforms with intention – transmitting consciousness through radiation to intended receivers. The effects of intention were illustrated by thirty years of research by Dr. Cleve Backster. Dr. Backster happened upon intentional communications in 1966 when he connected a dracaena plant to a polygraph machine. To his surprise, galvanic skin response readings from the equipment revealed that the plant responded to the potential of harm, specifically when there was an *intention to harm the plant*. This intention-sensing was found to also take place among fertilized chicken eggs and human leukocytes separated from their hosts. Human white blood cells kept *in vitro* sensed their hosts' emotion episodes (Backster, 2003).

In the same way that radios and televisions are tuned into the broadcasts of radio and TV stations, our bodies contain special cellular receptors specifically tuned to the informational waves of the sun. These receptors convert the sun's rays into heat, vitamin D and cellular processes we have yet to understand. Without the sun's informational waves, our bodies cannot function the way they were designed to function. Let's look at the science that supports this.

The Need for Sunlight

Over the past half century, researchers have been observing the effects of natural sunlight (or a lack thereof) upon plants, animals and humans. In the 1950s, while producing the famous Walt Disney time-lapse photography film, Dr. John Ott discovered that for flowering pumpkins grown indoors under fluorescent light, the male flowers would blossom but the female flowers would not. Meanwhile, outdoor pumpkins typically produce both male and female flowers.

Dr. Ott filmed and photographed flowers and plants indoors and outdoors. His time-lapse photography sessions with various flowers and plants revealed that plants without a full spectrum of infrared and ultraviolet light become, in one respect or another, disturbed. Dr. Ott's research on light and color continued into the 1980s and 1990s. He published numerous articles documenting his research – spanning over forty years – on the human body as well as plants and animals. These studies showed various negative effects resulting from a lack of natural sunlight upon the human body. They included mood disorders, learning disabilities, increased stress, abnormal growth, and poor eyesight among others. Without regular sunlight, humans – like plants – will begin to degenerate in a host of ways. As many of us have observed, should a plant be shut into a room with nothing but artificial light, its flowers and/or fruits will soon wilt and whither.

The effect of sunlight on animal and plant fertility has been known by farmers and ranchers for many years. The poultry and hog industries have known for years that full-spectrum light increases egg production and larger hog litters respectively. It has also been observed that human fertility also improves with sunbathing. We also know the increase in the warmth and duration of the sun stimulates the production of pollen and flowers among plants.

Dr. Ott's experiments with sunlight and rabbits revealed that rabbits raised under artificial light – especially among males – became more aggressive even to the point of becoming cannibalistic. Meanwhile, rabbits raised in sunlight showed none of these tendencies. Male rabbits raised in natural sunlight were not only less aggressive: They were also observed graciously tending to the litter in the absence of mama rabbit.

Humans are no exception. Significant research has established that not only do humans require light for health, but they require natural light. Several studies have found a link between fluorescent lights and hyperactivity among children (O'Leary 1978). Research performed by Küller and Laike (1998) in Sweden, has illustrated that fluorescent lighting powered with conventional ballasts increase stress and lower accuracy. This study, done on adults working in laboratory offices, found that conventional ballast fluorescent lighting increased (stressful) alpha wave activity among subjects.

A lack of natural sunlight will also disrupt the body's endocrine systems. German ophthalmology Professor Dr. Fritz Hollwich published a study in 1979 showing that subjects working under white fluorescent tube lighting for a period of time produced significantly higher levels of stress hormones such as adrenocorticortropic hormone and cortisol. He also found that full-spectrum or natural light lowered levels of these hormones, and lowered stress among the subjects. Dr. Hollwich's research was pivotal in the decision to ban white fluorescent bulbs from most German hospitals.

Other research has confirmed the need for natural sunlight. The necessity of natural light in an outdoor environment was established as a healing therapy by Azar and Conroy (1992). Camping had a therapeutic effect upon subjects attempting addiction recovery in Bennet et al. (1998). Bishop and Rohrmann (2003) illustrated how natural environments produced more positive subjective responses than simulated environments. Davis-Berman and Berman (1989) illustrated how adolescents were positively affected by wilderness settings. Freeman and Stansfield (1998) showed how urban environments create increased stress and anxiety. Gesler (1992) illustrated how natural geography affects medical disorders thera-peutically. Hammit (2000) illustrated that even an urban forest environment resulted in the reduction of stress and anxiety. As for the placement of windows and entrances, Heerwagen (1990) estab-lished that the size, design and placement of windows in a house had significant psychological effects upon those living in the house. Honeyman (1992) established that increased vegetation in the sur-rounding area significantly lowered stress levels. Kaplan (1983; 1992; 1992) also established that being surrounded by nature had positive psychological effects, increased well-being and significant positive behavioral responses. Pacione (2003) established that natu-ral landscapes even in an urban environment positively affects well-being. Dr. Robert Ulrich showed in over two decades of research that nature's landscapes, natural scenes, natural environments, and being surrounded by plants have a significant therapeutic effect (1979; 1981; 1983; 1984; 1992; 2002).

For some time it was assumed that *seasonal affective disorder* (SAD) relates only to the amount of light. However, this does not explain the lower levels of SAD among many northern climate cultures such as Eskimos as compared to lower latitude dwellers. SAD, as most know, is a serious disorder causing depression, anxiety, fatigue, and lethargy.

For example, a study from Iceland's National University Hospi-tal (Maqnusson and Stefansson 1993), found that Icelanders experience lower SAD prevalence than do people on the east coast of the United States. In another study from Turku University's Cen-tral Hospital (Saarijarvi *et al.* 1999), the prevalence of SAD was higher among women and younger ages, but notably also more prevalent among those with a higher body mass index. Higher BMI is also more likely among people who go outdoors less. There are many other studies indicating lower rates of SAD among those who exercise outdoors.

Indoor light ranges from 60 lux at low lamp level to 200 lux in average indoor lighting. The brightest indoor lighting might pro-duce about 1000 lux. Levels of over 1000 lux typically require some sort of daylight.

Light Intensity

Source of Light	Illumination Intensity (Lux)
Direct Sunlight	25,000-125,000 lux
Overcast day	100-20,000 lux
Daylight (out of sun)	7,000-13,000 lux
Sunrise and sunset	300-500 lux
Typical office lighting	200-400 lux
Typical home lighting (60-100W bulbs)	50-200 lux
Outdoor night (full moon/clear)	.25-1 lux
Outdoor night (1/4 moon)	.001 lux
Outdoor night (moonless/clear)	.002 lux
Sirius (brightest star)	.000001 lux

The typical American gets a few hundred lux per day on average, experiencing only quick bursts of a higher lux – likely barely over 1000 lux. 1000 lux is about as much light as is available in the twilight period – just after sunset or just before sunrise. Light above this level for three hours will re-establish sleep cycles and positive moods within 48 hours. Light greater than 4000 lux is needed for most endocrine-stimulating functions. Going outside into the sunlight is required for these levels.

Daily sunlight with dark nights is best. In a study of 1,606 women 20-74 years old (Davis *et al.* 2001), those who had either bright bedroom lights at night or worked graveyard shifts had higher breast cancer rates.

The research shows that those with consistent exposure to nature's visible light, ultraviolet light, infrared radiation and geomagnetism will be less likely to experience the depression, fatigue and other symptoms often experienced by those who spend their days inside amongst the artificial suns of our indoor world.

Natural Light Strategies

* **Windows are better:** If we cannot go outside, using natural window light is far better than indoor lighting. Keeping our windows unshaded throughout the day is therefore critical. Demand a window location from your employer. You can quote some of the research quoted here to prove that window lighting improves productivity among workers.

* **Look out:** If we are reading or working at our computer during the day – or otherwise working inside – we should consider looking out the window every few minutes.

* **Set up an outdoor living room and office:** Convenience often dictates habit. Setting up outdoor sitting and working areas will enable us to spend more time outside. Set up next to an outdoor outlet for outdoor computer work. Set up a table near the kitchen door to eat more meals outside.

* **Use sunglasses minimally:** Sunglasses block important light rays from reaching our eyes. They also polarize or diffract light. They mute color as well. Sunglasses can create a depressive state because they limit exposure of light to our pineal gland, changing our output of important energy and mood hormones and neurotransmitters (such as GABA, dopamine and serotonin). If we must wear sunglasses during driving or boating to prevent glare, they should be taken off periodically. Also, consider non-glare sunglasses that polarize with minimal darkening.

* **Choose indoor lights carefully:** Many indoor office and lighting systems have poor quality fluorescent lamps. Older models with conventional ballasts tend to flicker at lower frequencies. Their blinking will range from 60-100 times per second. The newer technology of high frequency electronic-ballast compact fluorescent light bulbs have increased frequencies in the 20-40 kilohertz range – over 2000 times faster than the older models. Higher-speed flickering seems to have a far less negative affect. These are recommended. Better is the 'full-spectrum' version.

* **Consider sun gazing:** Sun gazing during sunrise and sunset can have a rejuvenating effect upon the eyes if done correctly. Watching the sunset and sunrise has been a recommendation for eyesight problems among many traditional medicines including Ayurvedic, North American Indian, Mayan and Greek disciplines. The filtering of the earth's atmosphere during these two times of the day filters the rays considered damaging during the mid-day sun. Both

the ultraviolet and the infrared spectrum are almost completely blocked 15 minutes before the sunset and 15 minutes after sunrise. These times are typically safe to look directly at the sun. We can also check our local weather station website, the newspaper or the NOAA weather service for the hourly ultraviolet index.

* **Eyesight:** Consistent sunset/rise gazing every day can have the effect of improving eyesight. Many have reported seeing brighter colors. Many report a positive change in moods – a greater sense of optimism. Most report feeling relaxed and calm. The synchronizing effect between our SCN cells, pituitary, hypothalamus, and visual cortex can also lead to better sleep quality and a reduction in muscle tension. Evening or morning sunset/rise gazing is best done intermittently, accompanied by blinking and looking away at other natural images in the distance. Initially we can point the eyes and face at the setting or rising sun with eyes closed. After doing this for a few days, the eyes can gradually be opened, while blinking frequently – about once a second. After 10-15 seconds, the eyes can then wander over other images until the image of the sun has disappeared from the eyelids. As we progress over time, we can gradually repeat this process two or three times. Gazing at the setting or rising sun should always be accompanied with frequent blinking and looking away. During the first few weeks or months we can start with only a minute or two, gradually increasing to a comfortable 5-10 minutes. Consult with your eye specialist prior to undertaking gazing.

* **Meditate with the sun:** These two periods of the day – sunrise and sunset – have been considered crucial times for meditative processes by many faiths. Prayer, hymns, chanting and meditation are extremely effective at sunset and sunrise. These activities can be intermingled with the process of sunset/rise gazing as mentioned above, as we appreciate the consciousness pervading our universe.

* **Sunlight cautions:** It is not appropriate to stare at the sun 15 minutes after sunrise or fifteen minutes before sunset. If the sun is rising or setting upon the water this limit should be shortened to 10 minutes. Retinal damage can result if we stare at the sun when it is too high. This also applies to solar eclipses as well. Staring at a solar eclipse can damage our eyes as much as looking directly at the mid-day sun. We should also be careful looking at the sun while we are at higher altitudes or around water. At higher altitudes, there is less ozone and atmosphere available to filter ultraviolet. Because water reflects ultraviolet rays, sun intensity will be greater near the water.

* **Moon gazing and stargazing:** Moon gazing and stargazing are also helpful for eyesight, and can be meditative as well. Most of us have been awestruck by the beauty of the skies on a clear night. Finding that darkened place to spy at the distant galaxies, planets, and stars can provide us a view of that humbling expanse that is our universe. Focusing and unfocusing into the depths of space exercises the eyes. As in sun gazing, by peering in and out of the distances between and among the stars, our pupils enlarge and narrow, and along with it, our ciliary muscles, scleras, retinas, and zonular fibres all bend and flex with the changing focus. As we gaze, our eyes dart back and forth from star to star, the cavity of vitreous humour, optic disc and suspensory ligaments all adjust and resize with our focus. All of these motions help build strength into the eyes. In addition to these mechanical benefits, the informational electromagnetic wave content of the rays coming from the stars and galaxies benefits us in ways we have yet to understand.

* **Light therapy:** There are now a number of "full-spectrum" light devices on the market. Most are far better than typical indoor light. They don't replace the sun, but can be good for extreme northern locales or during extreme weather conditions. Research has shown that multiple hours a day are needed for therapeutic response. Look for 5,000 to 10,000 lux lamps. Read instructions carefully before use.

Chapter Four

Thermal Therapeutics

The ability of the sun to transfer thermal energy is not foreign to us. Most of us have sat down in a nice sun-warmed chair, or walked across a sun-heated beach. Most of us have also witnessed the heat inside a building in the summer, as the hot thermal waveforms of the sun beat down upon the materials of the outer walls of the building. This transfer of thermal radiation takes place as the infrared waveforms are exchanged from one molecule to the other throughout the building materials. This begins with the surface molecules and – depending upon the insulative or conductive nature of those molecular bonds – is transferred through to the inner layers of the material. If the molecules are good conductors of infrared waveforms, the summer sun will make the material too hot to touch. If the molecules have good insulating ability, the material will not feel very hot at all.

There are several ways materials may transfer thermal energy. Radiation is the most efficient transfer. This usually takes place through the atmosphere and through space, but it can also take place through other types of mediums, including water and some types of solids. Thermal waveforms may also be transferred through *conduction*. Conduction takes place when one molecule is hotter than its neighboring molecule. Thermal energy tends to flow from hotter to colder molecules through solids during conduction.

Thermal energy may also be transferred through *convection*. Convection is primarily the same action as conduction, but it takes place primarily within fluids. In convection, thermal energy tends to transfer from hotter molecules to cooler ones in an effort to equalize the thermal energy equally among the fluid.

As photosynthesis takes place within plants, a transfer of thermal energy also occurs. For example, hot climates appear to support the growth of botanicals that transfer thermal heat to spiciness. One of many examples is *capsicum sp.*, also called chili pepper or cayenne, which grows predominantly in hotter climates or higher altitudes. Chili peppers impart a heat that stimulates an increase in metabolism and immune function within the body. This in turn increases core body temperature, and assists the body to purge bacteria, which are also more prevalent in hotter climates.

This same effect is seen with *Piper nigrum* or black pepper, another hot climate plant. Black pepper is recommended by Ayurvedic physicians to increase *pitta* in the digestive tract, stimulating the flow of digestive enzymes and gastrin. This in turn tends to increase appetite, further protecting the body from bacterial infection from water and food. Other hot-weather botanicals that transfer thermal heat include *garlic, ginger, cumin,* and *paprika.* Each of these also has antibiotic and detoxifying properties.

For humans, plants and most animals, the sun's resonating energies deliver waveforms that balance core body temperature. Higher core body temperatures facilitate increased cell function and greater energy. This increases our metabolism, providing increased pathways for the body's various detoxification and purification systems. Boosted core temperatures increase cortisol levels during the day, which are balanced by increased melatonin levels – ushering greater relaxation and deeper sleep during the night.

While our body's temperature may be different at different locations at any particular point in time, our body core temperature typically must remain in a restricted range in order for our body to remain healthy. The typical core temperature of a healthy human body is about 98.2 degrees F, or 36.8 degrees C. This can range about a degree throughout the day and night. Even a slight reduction of body core temperature, such as occurs when we sleep, will significantly affect our metabolism. In fact, body core temperatures fluctuate slightly in a rhythmic fashion, similar to the sine wave motion of many of our other body rhythms.

Our body core temperature may not be reflected by our external sensations. For example, we may have a fever of several degrees, while our body core temperature may be on the low side. Often a fever simply reflects higher metabolism as our body's cells and processes are operating at higher levels of productivity.

The human body also radiates thermal energy. The human body radiates from about 100 to 500 watts continuously, depending upon the person's age, health, and metabolism. A younger, more active person will typically radiate thermal waveforms at a higher level. During intense activity, a person's body may radiate well over 500 watts of thermal heat. Hugging is a means of transferring this radiating heat from one person to another. As heat is transferred, the body will radiate and convect that heat. This becomes self-evident in a crowded room, bus, or rail car. As bodies fill the room, their radiating thermal energy increases the room temperature substantially. For this reason, we often see people sweating in a crowded bus or train, regardless of the temperature outside.

If the room temperature is cooler, the body will be working to maintain its core temperature. It will thus radiate less heat. If we were to chart the body's thermal radiation, we would also find a cyclical pattern evident. We would find that during the nighttime and during sleep, radiation heat decreases. It then increases dramatically in the morning – rising and falling through the day with the body's cortisol and thyroid hormone cycles. Typically, we find body temperatures gain through the morning – peaking and descending by around ten to eleven a.m. After dipping into the afternoon, body temperatures begin to rise substantially in the later afternoon. During these heightened periods – the morning and the later afternoon – humans tend to perform more activity. Many exercise during these higher morning and afternoon temperature cycles for this reason. After night falls, we begin to radiate less, as our core body temperature supports the lower metabolism of sleep.

Physical radiation cycles tend to be about 24-25 hours in period. There are other body thermal cycles to consider as well. Most mammals tend to produce more heat during the spring and fall. During these periods, core metabolism is up. During the peak of the summer solar cycle, the body will slow down to try to reduce heat. To reduce heat, the body's radiative thermal temperature will increase. In the winter, most mammals tend to get cozy in their hideaways, and perform less strenuous outdoor activity. Their metabolism tends to slow down and they tend to sleep more. Black bears, for example, slow down quite a bit. They sleep for long periods, and eat almost nothing during the winter. Though they do not completely hibernate as we used to think they did – sleeping the entire winter – they do indeed slow down quite a bit, and sleep more. During these 'down periods,' body heat is preserved, and radiative heat is thus reduced.

This cycling pattern of the physical body is not unlike the solar sunspot cycles of about every eleven years. During one part of the cycle, the sun's radiative thermal heat is reduced. During another part of the cycle, the sun's radiation of thermal heat is intensely increased. Could the sun's body be much different from our physical bodies? They both radiate thermal energy. They both undergo periodic cycling in their radiation periods. They both tend to have a birth and death – a definite lifespan. They both have periods of growth and periods of declination or aging. The nebula of a dying solar star is not unlike the graying and wrinkling of a once youthful physical body.

Radiant Matter

Radiant matter was first described by Sir William Crookes during his cathode ray experiments in the mid-nineteenth century. His research was updated in the late nineteenth century by Sir Joseph John Thomson using principles of subatomic matter.

Most of today's chemists and physicists will agree with the first three elemental states of matter – solids, liquids and gases. Every basic chemistry course and most physics curricula describe these three 'states' as forming the foundation of molecular matter. However, the ancient sciences go further, describing two additional elemental states. Various traditional sciences include *fire* or *heat* as a basic elemental state. While we know thermal energy can be derived from fire, fire is considered by today's science as a specific phenomena derived from the combustion of matter.

Thermal energy radiates from a source of atomic power. The sun is by far the largest source of thermal energy in our solar system and on our planet. The earth itself is a source of thermal energy, seemingly from an active core.

Like the sun and the earth, the human body also produces thermal radiation. This is the result of the life within the body. While the body is alive, it is actively stimulating metabolism. Metabolism produces heat through catalytic enzyme reaction. By far the most predominant reaction in the body is the metabolic conversion of glucose, oxygen, water and minerals to energy and heat.

The sun also utilizes atomic reactions to produce energy and heat. Research suggests that most of the sun's energy is produced through nuclear fusion. This is a process whereby the nuclei of two hydrogen proton atoms come together to form helium. Energy and heat are created as byproducts.

Like the earth, much of the sun's thermal energy is seemingly produced within its core. The theory is that the proton fusion within the core is taking place at an incredible rate, and this pushes the kinetic energy outward, driving more fusion towards the surface. This theoretically produces the high-energy gamma rays, infrared rays, and many other EMF waves. This core is also thought to be the source of the biomagnetism that is being produced by the sun.

Thermal radiation moves through matter, speeding up or slowing down molecular movement, which results in a change of temperature and structure. In another perspective, we could conclude that solids contain the quality of shape, liquids contain the quality of flow, and gases contain the quality of pressure. Likewise, thermals contain the quality of temperature.

Thermals typically radiate within the infrared waveforms, although thermals also can be transferred through visible, microwave, ultraviolet and x-ray radiation as well. Infrared waves also have a spectrum of waveforms. The infrared region is typically divided between several wavelength types: *Near infrared* waveforms are closer to visible light with a shorter wavelength of about .7 to one micrometers in wavelength. *Short-wave infrared* waveforms range from about one to three micrometers. *Mid-wave infrared* waves range from three to five micrometers. *Long-wave infrared* waves range from about seven to fourteen micrometers. *Far infrared* radiation ranges from about 15 to about 1,000 micrometers in wavelength. Infrared radiation produces thermal heat by interfering with (or "exciting") the bonding waveforms of molecules they come into contact with.

Just as do the other elemental states, waveform interference can alter the state of a group of molecules. Should we apply a Bunsen burner onto a flask of chemicals, we will quickly change those chemicals from one state to another. Thermal radiation thus provides a catalyst for change. Anytime we blend one type of elemental state with another, the same response results: A characteristic change in the character of one or more of the substances. In the example mentioned above, bubbling a gas through a liquid will generally result in a molecular alteration of both the liquid and the gas. The liquid will pick up various molecules available in the gas, and the gas will be affected by the liquid. In the same way, if we allow water to encounter a solid, we will observe some of the solid dissolving into the water. The water's chemistry will change and the solid area will be eroded by the water.

The orbital bonds of molecules are altered during thermal heat conduction. This can cause electrons to jump to higher energy orbitals, releasing heat. This is the result of waveform interference between the bonds and the infrared radiation.

This change in atomic orbital states provides a precise mechanism for metabolism. Thermal energy production stimulates the catalytic processes that drive metabolism. It is metabolism that renders our bodies the ability to move, function and produce heat.

Radiation can be either inhibitory or effective. An inhibitory radiative response may increase skin temperature, but it may not significantly raise body core temperature. Typically, an alternating current heat source like electrical heat will result in an inhibitory response. This will create stress in the body. It may yield a slightly increased body core temperature, but part of this results from the inhibitory response, which is comparable to an inflammatory response. Heat from alternating current is not receptive because the body's epidermal and dermal cellular receptors are designed for the thermal waveforms from the sun, fire, earth or other living organisms. These sources of radiation provide constructive interference.

Any sort of stressor or toxicity within the body will typically result in an increase in thermal output, as the body increases metabolism to purge the unwelcome visitor. After the cleansing, body temperature should fall quickly, helping to rebalance the body's cellular homeostasis. In this way, a fever should not be seen as a disorder or ailment. Rather, it is part of the process of cleansing. Without increased thermal activity, our bodies would be overburdened with toxicity.

Within nature's ecosystem, thermal changes result in similar mechanisms of homeostasis, but with a lower stress response. This is why a plant might remain healthy in 100 degrees F of sun exposure, but shrivels when put close to a 100-degree electric heater. The human body is the same way. Our cells were designed to respond appropriately to the heat of the sun.

The entire ecosystem is tuned to the thermal radiation of the sun and earth. As the warmer waters of the ocean are evaporated and move through wind and storm systems, an upwelling of colder water brings nutrients to the surface. This temperature conveyor system cycles nutrients throughout the oceans and water over the land.

This mechanism is also prevalent among various closed biosystems. In the late eighteenth and early nineteenth century, Henry Le Chatelier observed and documented this effect. He observed particular chemical reactions responding to stressors. The result of the reactions reduced the influence of the stressor. This law became known as *Le Chatelier's Principle*.

The sun produces around half the thermal energy existing within our environment. Other sources of thermal energy are the various living organisms, the earth (another living organism), and reflective thermal energy resulting from various types of waveform interactions. The human organism produces a substantial amount of thermal radiation, as we have discussed. The human body and related mammals apparently radiate thermal energy in the wavelength range of about ten microns.

Nerve-endings within our skin cells are sensitive to thermal energy being radiated from other elements. When these skin nerve receptors – better thought of as *antennas* – pick up the waveforms of infrared waves, they translate and send signals through the central nervous system to the brain and cognitive centers. These signals allow the neural network to respond to the thermal input. Waveforms out of context with the ecosystem are interpreted as stressful and potentially harmful. This produces the burning sensation.

On a cellular basis, the thermal elemental state produces various coherent wave structures, which can result in a combination of conduction, convection, and/or simple radiation. These waveform effects allow thermal heat to circulate within the body through a network of subtle energy channels.

In Chinese medicine, the circulation of thermal energy plays an important role in the diagnosis of illness. Just as liquids circulate through blood vessels, the Chinese determined that thermals circulate through subtle channels called *meridians*. These channels have gateways, which increase or reduce the flow of heat. For example, a Chinese medical doctor might determine through examination that a person has excess heat in the liver. Acupuncture treatment will 'drain' this heat from the liver by applying needles to the gateways in order to interfere with the heat circulation. The process, controlled by the expertise of a well-trained acupuncturist, in effect pulls heat away from that part of the body.

European and western medicine has also long respected the relationship between thermal energy and health. For this reason, thermometers are used extensively to measure one's wellness. Temperature is also used to estimate ovulation timing. Depending upon the person's metabolism, during ovulation the basal temperature will typically rise about a degree Fahrenheit. Basal temperature is also a strong indicator of the health of the thyroid gland. Low morning basal temperature is associated with suppressed thyroid gland function. Temperature increases at local sites are also often associated with fighting an infection or healing an injury at the site. Inflammation is a widely recognized symptom of an active immune response among all medical disciplines.

Increases in thermal radiation can directly affect waveform energy levels within impacted molecules. This can interfere with the subatomic bonds within the atoms of the molecule. A molecule that has been so damaged is imbalanced, and needs to re-establish its sub-atomic balance by stealing sub-atomic parts from other molecules. This can produce what is called a *radical*. Radicals are highly reactive molecules or ions that have unbalanced bonding orbitals. This imbalance produces a situation where the radical needs to steal or share bonding orbitals with another molecule or atom.

This is also seen when thermal radiation cooks food: When water and food is heated with thermal radiation, the atoms and molecules in the food and water become more active due to their respective bonding orbitals being boosted to new frequencies. This increase results in the water's boiling and the food's cooking. Water conducts this thermal radiation. The radiation is carried through the molecules of water, analogous to light diffracting and refracting through water. While not precisely the same mechanism, the radiation is passed around from atom to atom as bonds are disturbed. Thermal radiation disturbs the bonding energy states, which slowly changes the shape and condition of the food. As the food is cooked in the water, the radiation being passed through the water alters the bonds of the molecules in the food, making the food more chewable. This is accompanied by a loss of heat-sensitive nutrients.

The sun's thermal radiation is also being conducted through the medium of space, then the atmosphere and finally, through our bodies. If we were to look at a large flame of fire burning in a fireplace, for example, we would immediately notice there is not just one large round flame. Instead, there are thousands of little flickering flames, jumping up and down. As these little flames pop up and down, they continually push out radiation as they flame up. Once they flare up, they will merge back into the fire to become indistinguishable. These flames crackle noisily as they pierce the air in reach of oxygen and combustible fuel.

Are these little flames subunits of the larger fire just as electrons are considered subunits of atoms? Similar to atoms and electrons, the flames are difficult to locate, yet they encircle the core fire. Yet should we try to capture any particular flame and separate it from the fire, we will certainly become frustrated. Either we will end up with a separate fire with new flames to contend with, or we would snuff out that part of the fire.

As we consider the various sources of heat on this planet carefully, it becomes obvious that our sun is the primal source of all heat. The sun is the source for the nutrients that we gain from food. As we convert the plant-sugars created through photosynthesis, we are indirectly processing the sun's energy into our own heat. If we consider the earth's thermal core, we can connect the sun with the earth's existence. The sun maintains the earth's ecosystems, allowing the earth's conveyer systems to utilize carbon to maintain its below-surface operations. Even the heat generated by fire or carbon burning is directly attributable to the sun's conversion of plant matter.

The ancient Vedic and Chinese sciences pointed out thousands of years ago that the thermal state is related to digestion, physical activity, metabolism, war, violence, passion, and anger. Ayurvedic tradition also says the thermal elemental state is specific to conversion, biodegradation, energy, change, vision, destruction, and metabolism. Its ability to stimulate energy conversion makes it essential for living organisms. Thermals are also considered cleansing. It is no coincidence that equipment is sterilized using thermal radiation. Heat damages pathogenic microorganisms through overheating. It also speeds up just about every metabolic process – including detoxification and nerve conduction.

The sun's thermal waveforms combine as they collide with our body to effect this increased metabolism. The body's absorption of the sun's full-spectrum of radiation stimulates a complex metabolic response.

Part of this complex response was shown in a study of peripheral neuropathy conducted by researchers from the Veterans Affairs Northern California Division (Swislocki *et al.* 2009). One hundred and twenty-one patients with painful diabetic peripheral neuropathy were given either photon stimulation (thermal light therapy) or placebo treatments. Among the group receiving the photon treatments, 28% reported a slight reduction in pain while 34% reported a moderate reduction in pain after only four treatments. We should note that peripheral neuropathy is a very complex and difficult pain condition to treat.

Heat is critical for healthy metabolism. Heat relaxes the artery walls, which increases circulation. This in turn speeds the transfer of nutrients, plasmin, lymphocytes and other elements that travel the bloodstream. As these elements are delivered to body tissues, they can influence the health of that tissue faster. Increased circulation will also speed the removal of toxins and broken down molecular parts. As these are removed, the body is able to repair damage and regenerate tissue.

Thermal Strategies

* **Heat therapy:** The sun's thermal heat can be very helpful during bouts of fever or chills. During fever, the sun's heat promotes sweating and detoxification. During chills, the sun's heat raises body core temperature. The sun's thermals can support healing mechanisms for many illnesses, and can increase immunity to prevent illness.

* **Saunas:** Many use saunas to heat the body and speed up healing. Traditional saunas used fires and hot stones in an outdoor environment such as a tent. North American Indians have used sweat lodges, and the Finnish used fired furnaces in this fashion. Modern versions usually include a wooden room with an electric heating filament, some with

hot stones for pouring water. Saunas are an effective way to increase healing times and detoxification.

* **The modern filament sauna** is the least desirable, because the dry alternating current output heats up the dermal layer faster than the epidermal layers and inner tissues. This imbalance in heat can stress the body. For this reason, this type of sauna can cause dizziness, fainting and urgent cardiovascular events. Used with caution, this sauna can still successfully produce detoxification, however.

* **The sweat lodge** is a wonderful sauna strategy because it is outdoors, and utilizes the natural thermal radiation from fire, which heats the body more gradually and internally. Care must be taken to keep fire smoke out of the lodge, however. Smoke inhalation can be deadly. To make a sweat lodge, simply dig a fire pit and begin a fire with some larger, easy-to-lift stones sitting close to the fire. Erect a small building frame or teepee close by, using sticks from the surrounding environment if possible. In the middle of the framework, dig a small pit and cover pit and ground inside with sage or similar aromatic plants from surrounding area (eucalyptus is nice too). Drape some heavy blankets over the frame. Place rocks at the bottom ends to seal the lodge. After the fire has gone on for a few hours, the stones will be sufficiently hot. Find a sturdy cloth or piece of wood to roll the hot (not fiery) stones onto, and carry into the covered lodge. Enclose the lodge. With ten large stones or more smaller stones, the lodge should get nice and hot.

* **The far infrared sauna** provides a great form of thermal therapy during colder winter weather. It is good for chronic pain, fatigue, congestion, muscle aches and certainly for over-toxicity. Because it improves circulation, the infrared sauna stimulates the body's healing response. This is because the infrared waveforms more easily pierce through our dermal and epidermal layers, immediately expanding blood vessels and micro-capillaries to stimulate healing, relax muscles and soothe nerves. This immediate effect is

quite noticeable, and for this reason, infrared saunas, and infrared massage tools have become extremely popular and effective for detoxification and stimulating circulation. The far-infrared system uses a series of infrared lamps placed around the sauna room to heat the skin directly. A cool or cold bath after any sauna can additionally serve to stimulate the immune system, improve cardiovascular function, and increase lymphatic circulation. Increased water intake is vital during and directly following any sauna. It is best to take at least a half-gallon of water into any sauna.

* **The sun sauna:** The sun, of course, emits the best infrared radiation. The sun's infrared radiation is tuned to the body's cells. Therefore, the specific waveforms of the sun's thermal infrared waves resonate deeply with the body, opening up micro-capillaries and tissue systems. There is little resistance or stress from the body during heating by the sun. An infrared sauna may also have detoxifying infrared waveforms, but these will accompany subtle electromagnetic waveforms that are a product of alternating current – a modified or synthetic waveform.

* **To make a sun sauna:** The sun sauna simply consists of sitting outside in the direct mid-day sun with a hat, comfortable cotton or wool sweat pants and sweatshirt – allowing the body to sweat by trapping the sun's thermal radiation within the clothing. A hot summer's day is optimal for an outdoor sun sauna, but a sun sauna can work during any season's afternoon sun. In cooler temperatures, simply put on more clothes until sweating is accomplished. Wearing gloves and lightly binding the edges of the clothing around the neck, arms and ankles will help more completely trap the heat within the clothing. Sun saunas can also be done with tents or sunrooms. A cloth army tent or other thick material tent that blocks ultraviolet is recommended to make the sun tent. A ventilated woodshed can also make a nice sun sauna room.

* **Extremity sunning:** Letting the warmth of the sun's thermal rays strike our feet and legs increases microcirculation, especially useful in areas of the body where capillaries and blood vessels weaken with age. The effects of the sun's thermal radiation can increase venous circulation and organ health. In addition, we can walk barefoot on an earthen surface heated by the sun. This might include warm beach sand, grass, or even better, large smooth rocks heated by the sun. The thermal waveforms stored within these elements will radiate up through the soles of our feet, delivering the sun's thermal effects deep into our body core.

* **Daily thermals:** Obtaining thermal energy from the sun on a daily basis is essential. When the sun comes up, our bodies need the sun's thermal radiation to maintain many of our metabolic functions. As the day pulses on, we increasingly find that our core body temperature relates directly to our radiative environment. A constant indoor environment leads to slower metabolism and a colder core body temperature. This especially holds true during colder weather or changing weather. Daily infrared radiation exposure will increase enzyme activity and improve cognition.

* **IR therapy:** A number of infrared ("light therapy") massage devices are available. These are incredible ways to relax muscles, increase microcirculation and stimulate healing.

* **Finding balance:** Establishing a balanced core temperature requires us to seasonally make adjustments between sun and shade, and indoor and outdoor activities. These adjustments provide rhythm and balance to our activities. As we cyclically adjust with the seasons and outdoor time, we will be synchronizing our body to nature's cycles. To test and discover our thermal balance, a digital oral thermometer is suggested for accuracy. Readings are best taken after resting periods only, such as upon waking or after sitting for a while. Temperature is optimal between 97.9 and 98.6. Try for a few days each season with a diary several times during the day to establish body core temperature cycles. This can

be extremely useful for someone with low energy, chronic fatigue or chronic pain. If body temperature is more than 1 degree F low in the morning, sleep quality and/or thyroid hormones should be suspected. Report this to your physician. Low thyroid hormones can be problematic.

* **Creating thermal balance** is quite simple. This might consist merely of taking a daily walk through a natural environment of trees and meadows, or working outside in the garden daily. During the hot summers, we can walk under trees or in the morning to be partially shaded and cooled. By walking in and out of the trees or as the sun begins to rise into the sky, we fall into a rhythm of alternating sun with intermittent shade. During the cooler winter months, we can seek more direct sunlight and less shade – the trees will help as many will have lost their leaves.

* **Location, Location:** Everything goes better with thermal heat. We can find a location in almost any building that has windows where we can soak up thermal rays from the sun. We need to be careful of exposing skin to direct window sun for too long, however. Glass blocks much of the UV-B rays while letting in unbalanced UV-A rays – which can cause skin damage. The thermal rays are still beneficial, however. Simply limit direct skin exposure. The best solution if it is not too cold outside is to simply open the window, or go outside to sit in the sun.

* **Degassing:** The sun can also be used to degas new materials we buy that contain preservatives, cements or other chemical additives. Many store-bought materials will be fumigated or covered in formaldehyde, for examples. Chemicals such as formaldehyde can be extremely toxic. New items with these types of chemicals should be degassed in the sun for a day or two before bringing them inside the house or otherwise becoming exposed to them. To degas, simply put the object out in the direct sunlight for a full day or two. The sun should significantly evaporate the toxins in most cases. Let the product stand in the cool shade

before bringing back in the house. To degas a new car's interior, simply let the car sit in the hot sun with the windows down for several days. Try not to drive the car with the windows up for a few weeks thereafter.

* **Solar ovens** are a great way to cook. These are actually quite simple to use, although they take more time than a conventional oven. A solar oven will require about three times the amount of time to bake something, given a hot sunny climate. The result, however, will be a great tasting dish that has retained a higher percentage of its nutrient content. For a simple solar oven, fill a large stainless steel or glass pot with food and water and lay it in direct sunlight. Mirrors or foil can be placed around the pot to increase cooking temperature.

* **Sun tea** is a great way to absorb the sun's thermals while making delicious herbal tea. Just put some herb leaves from the garden into a large glass jar or pitcher, and seal it with a small gap for air. Set the jar in direct sun for 2-3 hours in the mid-day, or for 3-4 hours in the sun during winter or other times of the day.

* **Solar water heaters** are efficient forms of household hot water production. Solar water heaters reduce our dependence upon carbon energy, while delivering water resonating with solar thermal waveforms.

* **Solar electricity:** Let's not forget the use of solar panels for generating electricity. There are now many different options, large and small, to produce power from the sun. Consider reducing the use of atmosphere-robbing carbon-based power by erecting solar panels for the home and office.

* **Sun foods:** Raw whole plant foods conduct thermal radiance through colorful phytonutrients. Spicy foods such as peppers, and sweet or sour fruits such as fruits will contain more thermal heat capacity than bitter foods. Within the body, these foods drive metabolism and increase body core temperature. While sweet and sour foods tend to encourage

greater energy output, spicy foods tend to stimulate circulation and detoxification.

* **Thermal stones:** A great way to absorb thermal radiance is using hot thermal stones. This is an ancient method used by the Polynesians (called *lomi lomi*), by North American Indians and by Ayurvedic practitioners (called *shila abhyanga*). These therapies typically utilize smooth flatter, hand-sized stones. The stones can be heated in hot water and applied to the skin after a little cooling. They are often applied with massage oil to penetrate heat deep into the skin. A better (and safer) approach is to heat the stones in the mid-day sun for an hour or two. The stones will more easily be handled, and can be applied to the skin more readily (still they should be cooled enough to handle). Massage oil can be used. The stones can also be laid directly onto the skin without oil.

* **Thermal balance:** Maintaining thermal seasonality is critical to metabolic and immune system homeostasis (balance). Today, most of us have air conditioners and heaters on practically all the time. These devices keep our bodies from resonating with nature's thermal waveforms. These devices also reduce our body's ability to naturally keep itself cooler in the summer and warmer in the winter. They also reduce our outdoor time and fresh air, as we shut ourselves in to keep in the heat or cold. Air conditioners should be used only when heat is intolerable. Otherwise, fans, cooling with water, and sweating (an efficient cooling and detoxification method) are better for our immune system. When driving, we can open the windows to let the wind through to cool us. We can also take cool showers to reduce our body core temperatures. In the winters, we can wear additional clothing, cuddle up with our significant others, use fire heat and utilize sunlight. These forms of heat do not stress the body, as do electric heaters or heat pumps using duct systems – likely teeming with mold and bacteria. Using nature's heating and cooling systems to the extent possible will strengthen the body's ability to adapt, thereby strengthening our immune system.

Chapter Five

Synthetic Sun

Most of us living in the modern world have replaced the sun with a synthetic version: electromagnetically driven lights and appliances. Modern humankind has harnessed electromagnetic radiation in the form of alternating current. For thousands of years, humans used the light of the sun as the primary means for observation and lifestyle. Fire, of course, augmented the sun at night. As any candlelight dinner will attest, the light given off by flame is a significantly different experience than today's fluorescent or incandescent lights.

Together, these two energy sources – sun and fire – provided the primary means of light and heat. Today these have been replaced by an electronic light show with innumerable blinking lights and pulsing electronics. Today's environment is drowning in supercharged alternating currents.

The question is, are there any negative health consequences from this replacement of energy? Does the synthetic surging of alternating current create negative effects upon our bodies and/or minds as compared to those currents driven by sun and fire?

We have addressed some of the issues of using artificial lights and sun tanning beds elsewhere. In our discussion of the sun's rhythmicity, we illustrated the research showing that artificial lights of even 100 lux can throw off the body's natural entrainment to the sun. The intrusion of artificial light has been shown to disrupt sleep cycles, increase stress and change hormone balance. Each of these effects, in turn, has negative consequences. Sleep, for example, is vital to practically every metabolic process and cognitive process in the body. Without a consistent pattern of enough sleep, our bodies can fall prey to mental stress and physical illness. Stress is known to be a causative or contributing factor in almost every illness. Hormone disruption can cause a variety of other metabolic problems, ranging from inflammation to pain.

In the sections on natural light and color, we discussed how sunlight produces, reflects and refracts a balance of waveforms that stimulate particular hormones and mood cycles. The research has shown that without natural light we will experience greater levels of stress, anxiety and even anger. The replacement of artificial light with sunlight has, in a number of studies, been shown to increase cognition, learning, and development among children. Among adults, natural sunlight increases memory and positive moods. Full-spectrum lighting has been shown to provide some of these effects. However, we should point out that it will be unlikely that human-kind will ever be able to reproduce the entire electromagnetic spectrum of the sun. As discussed, the sun produces a host of different waveforms with a precisely coherent balance.

In our sun medicine section, we will also discuss briefly how synthetic sun tanning bed lights can provide a mix of UV-A and UV-B that stimulates vitamin D production in the body. The downside is that these lights have also been shown to produce higher levels of cancers such as melanoma. The reason made obvious, once again, is that we have yet to reproduce all of the sun's balance of waveforms in the right proportion. In other words, our bodies are *tuned* to the total spectrum of electromagnetic radiation produced by the sun.

Today we have enclosed our bodies inside an environment of synthetic alternating electromagnetic radiation (EMR), effectively shielding or dampening the sun's natural radiation. Is this development a healthy one?

It has been assumed that, outside of electrocution, alternating current had little or no negative effects upon the body. Then about two decades ago, a sounding alarm was made. A plethora of research and documentation offered the possibility of negative effects from EMR. A controversial and embattled thesis arose: Perhaps electromagnetic radiation from alternating current creates unhealthy effects upon the body.

The primary question – taking up our focus – posed whether and to what degree electromagnetic radiation from alternating current sources causes cancer. Yes, this is an important question, but not the only important question. Equally important is to what extent electromagnetic radiation from alternating currents may affect our vitality and general wellness. Does it burden our immune system? Does it deplete our energy? Does it slow cognition? These questions have been curiously missed in much of the debate and research on EMR.

Today's environment is embedded with a plethora of electromagnetic pulses our bodies have never faced. We are surrounded by electronic appliances that emit varying degrees of electronic and magnetic field strength. Our buildings are wired with EMR-emitting circuits and breaker systems. Most of us spend multiple hours in front of computers and televisions, absorbing magnetic fields. The battery and transmission systems built into our phones, music players and laptops bring our skin in direct contact with EMR-emitting appliances.

With billions of us partaking in at least some of these activities daily without obvious negative effects, some wonder what all the fuss is about, and why some health proponents are still arguing the case against synthetic EMRs.

There are two basic forms of radiation to consider: *Ionizing radiation* and *non-ionizing radiation*. According to a 2005 report by the National Academy of Sciences on low levels of ionizing radiation, about 82% of America's ionizing radiation comes from natural sources: the earth, sun, space, food and the air. The rest – 18% – comes from human origin. The bulk of this fabricated radiation comes from x-rays and nuclear medicine. This accounts for close to 80% of the 18%. Other elements like consumer goods, toxic water, occupational exposure, and nuclear power account for the rest of the ionizing radiation exposure according to this report.

Ionizing Radiation

Ionizing radiation is typically defined as electromagnetic radiation capable of disrupting atomic, molecular or biochemical bonds. This disruption takes place through an interference of waveforms between the ionizing radiation and the waveforms of atomic or molecular orbital bonds. As this interference is likely to cause the atom or molecule to lose electrons, ions are likely to develop as a result. These ions can often turn to oxidative species or otherwise imbalanced molecular species. Should ionizing radiation with enough intensity impact the physical body, it can result in cell injury or mutagenic damage. Various natural and synthetic radiation forms are considered ionizing. Natural ionizing radiation includes portions of ultraviolet radiation, x-rays, cosmic rays and gamma rays. Fire can also cause ionizing radiation at high temperatures if the radiation comes close enough. Synthetic versions of ionizing radiation include electrically produced x-rays, CAT-scans, mass accelerator emissions and a host of other electromagnetic radiation produced through alternating current.

Non-ionizing radiation also can be split into natural and synthetic versions. Natural versions include sound, light and radiowaves. Most natural non-ionizing radiation can also be synthetically produced. For example, sound may be digitally produced through the manipulation of alternating current by stereo receivers and speakers. This effect utilizes electrical semiconduction. Some scientists also categorize radiation from electrical power lines, electricity generating or transfer stations, appliances, cell phones, cell towers and other shielded electricity currents as non-ionizing radiation. Microwaves are also considered non-ionizing. Most assume that non-ionizing radiation is not harmful. This assumption, however, has undergone debate over the past few decades.

The 2005 National Academy of Sciences report, after a review of most of the available research regarding non-ionizing radiation, concluded that even low doses below 100 milliseiverts were potentially harmful to humans and could cause a number of disorders from solid cancer or leukemia. This jolted the scientific community, because for many years researchers thought that small doses of non-ionizing radiation were not that harmful.

A rem is one unit of radiation dose in roentgens. The mrem is one thousandth of a rem. One hundred rem equals one sievert. One sievert equals one thousand milliseiverts. Ten sieverts (10,000 mSv) will cause immediate illness and death within a few weeks. One to ten sieverts will cause severe radiation sickness, and the possibility of death. Above 100 mSv there is a probability of cancer, and 50 mSv is the lowest dose that has been established as cancer causing. Twenty mSv per year has been established as the limit for radiological workers. About one to three mSv per year is the typical background radiation received from natural sources, depending upon our location and surroundings. About .2 to .7 mSv per year comes from air. Soil sources are responsible for about .8 mSv. Cosmic rays give off about .22 mSv per year. Japanese holocaust victims received .1 Sv to 5 Sv from the bomb.

Our total radiation dose is a thus a combination of natural sources and those emitted by our artificial electromagnetic empire. A report from the Hiroshima International Council for Health Care of the Radiation-Exposed noted that the world's average radiation dose from natural radiation sources is 2.4 mSv. However, they also noted that Japan's natural radiation average is comparably low at 1.2 mSv. Japan's average radiation dose from medical radiation is higher than average, at 2.4 mSv. This gives Japan a significantly higher radiation average of 3.6 mSv.

UK's National Radiological Protection Board estimates that the national radiation exposure in Britain for the average person is 2.6 mSv, with an estimated 50% coming from radon gas, 11.5% coming from foods and drinks, 14% coming from gamma rays, 10% coming from cosmic rays and 14% originating from appliances – primarily medical equipment.

Recent research indicates that radiation from medical equipment is increasing. This is primarily driven by the growing use of CT scans, which generate a larger dose of radiation than the more traditional x-rays. About sixty-two million CT scans are now given a year in the U.S., as opposed to about three million per year in 1980. Brenner and Hall (2007) reported in the *New England Journal of Medicine* that a third of CT scans given today are unnecessary. The article also estimated that between one and two percent of all cancers are caused by CT scan radiation exposure.

In contrast, the maximum radiation a nuclear electricity generating plant will emit at the perimeter fence is about .05 mSv per year. A set of dental x-rays will render a dose of about .05-.1 mSv. A CT scan can render a dose of about 10 mSv – over a hundred times the dose of an x-ray.

A grand electromagnetic human self-experiment is unfolding. Unsuspecting humans and animals are the subjects of this experiment. The findings will be available in a decade or two from now.

Most researchers are quick to say gamma rays – from radon and other natural sources – produce significantly more radiation than do appliances. This might be true for someone with a minimal amount of electrical appliances who rarely visits the hospital and dentist's office.

The question that persists is whether humankind's synthetic "non-ionizing radiation" is as innocuous as is currently assumed.

Power Lines

The American Physical Society, an association of 43,000 physicists, said in a 1995 National Policy (95.2) statement, *"....no consistent significant link between cancer and power line fields...."* This statement was reaffirmed by the APS council in April of 2005.

Power lines emit electromagnetic radiation at ELF or *extra low frequency* levels. Power lines typically release about 50 hertz of pulsed radiation. As an electric current moves through a wire or appliance, magnetic fields move perpendicular with electricity in a cross pattern. Thus, electricity fields form from the strength of the voltage while magnetic fields rise and break away from the electronic waveform's motion. While electricity voltage can shock us or burn the body, magnetic fields have more subtle yet lasting influences upon the body's natural biowave systems – such as brainwaves, neurotransmitter release, hormone production, and so on.

While magnetic influences are difficult to perceive directly, it is apparent they may substantially interrupt our immune systems. Between 1970 and 2000, about fourteen international studies analyzed the potential link between power lines and cancer among children. Eight of those studies showed a link between cancer rates and power line proximity, while four studies associated power lines with leukemia.

One of the U.S. studies to show a positive link in between cancer took place in 1979 in Denver, led by Dr. Nancy Wertheimer and Ed Leeper. This studied showed a more than double likelihood of cancer among children living within forty meters of a high-voltage line. Another Denver study published in 1988 (Savitz *et al.*) also found a 1.54x odds ratio (OR) positive link in all childhood cancers and high power lines. A Danish study (Olsen *et al.* 1993) also linked general cancer rates (1.5 OR) with power line proximity. A study done in Los Angeles (London *et al.* 1991) showed a 2.15 OR rate, a Swedish study (Feychting and Ahlbom 1992) showed a 3.8 OR risk and a Mexican (Fajardo-Gutierrez *et al.* 1993) study showed 2.63 OR increased rate of leukemia cancer rates among children with close proximity to high-voltage power lines. One Swedish study (Tomenius 1986) showed a 3.7 OR increased risk for central nervous system tumors among children living close to power lines. The

Danish study mentioned above also showed a 5.6 OR increased potential of all cancers among children. The other positive link studies showed rates above 1 to 1.5 OR, which are not considered by mainstream science to be statistically significant.

Following the release of these studies, a number of governments took steps to warn housing developers of the potential risks of building close to high frequency power line hubs. In some municipalities across Europe and the U.S., building departments have even taken steps to dissuade or ban developments close to larger power lines.

Adult power line studies have yet to illustrate as large a correlation between power line proximity and cancer rates. Still a few have been significant enough to confirm the need for concern. Werthheimer and Leeper's (1982) studies showed increased rates of all cancers. Still, this 1.28 OR rate was not considered that significant. However a U.K. study (McDowall 1986) showed a SMR 215 increased rate of lung cancer and a SMR 143 increased risk (SMR 100 or less = no risk) of leukemia. Another study in the U.K (Youngson 1991) showed a statistically insignificant 1.29 OR rate for leukemia and lymphoma and Feychting and Ahlbom's (1992) Swedish study showed a 1.7 OR risk for leukemia subtypes. Another significant study (Schreiber *et al.* 1993) showed a SMR=469 rate for Hodgkin's disease.

It must be noted that these studies are epidemiological. They are population studies where groups living in close-proximity to high frequency power lines are compared with groups living further away. The problems that can occur with these studies focusing on cancer are several. In cancer pathology, there can be a two to twenty year delay between exposure and cancer diagnosis. While some of the populations involved in these studies might have been living in a particular house for many years, most may have only lived there for a year or two at the most.

In addition, some of the studies limited the disease group population, restricting the usefulness of the information. Cancer is seen primarily in the elderly and middle-aged, where there may be a host of various different types of exposures. These would include smoking, alcohol consumption, job-related exposures, chemical toxins, and so on. For this reason, these studies can be difficult to weigh against the costs of preventing exposure. The economic issues involving power lines are quite substantial. Relocating schools and families away from high-voltage lines or even relocating power lines comes with a substantial economic cost.

Nonetheless, this is increasingly becoming a problem for both homeowners and utility companies. For example, in the mid-nineties, the New Jersey Assembly enacted legislation requiring disclosure from homebuilders of vicinity transmission lines in excess of 240 kilovolts (kV). Other states have followed with real estate disclosure laws for power lines. Lawsuits have followed on power line proximity issues between schools, buyers, builders and utility companies.

One of the problems existing with some of the power line studies is the comparable limits of the distances between households and power lines. For example, is the effect of a transformer 40 meters away significantly different from one 50 meters away? Another difficulty with these epidemiological power line studies is that some of the studies measured utility wire codes (wire thickness) and distance, while other studies used spot physical measurements to determine exposure levels. In addition, there has been a variance of controls related to whether the child was born in the house or moved there recently.

With regard to the significance of the leukemia studies, we should consider the incidence of leukemia cancer among the childhood population – close to 1 in 10,000. A 2 or 3 OR among a group, unless the size of the groups are in the millions (most of the studies were significantly smaller – in the thousands), would relate to only a small handful of disease cases over the entire study population. If the study group size was five or ten million, then these numbers might be considered more reliable. As the increased rates have been smaller (rather than the 4 or 5 OR rate that appears in many study groups) then the size of the disease group is not considered to be a significant factor with which to judge the quality of the study. To this point, D'Arcy Holman, a professor at the University of Western Australia, calculated that the UK studies' worst projections might mean one extra childhood leukemia death in Western Australia every fifty years (Chapman 2001).

Occupational studies regarding exposure to EMR have shown unclear results with regard to leukemia and cancer (Kheifets *et al.* 2008). However, studies have pointed to the increased risk of amyotrophic lateral sclerosis (ALS) due to EMR exposure (Johansen 2004). Studies on electricians, electric utility line workers and other electrical workers have consistently showed higher rates of leukemia and central nervous system-related cancers. In a 2006 meta-study of fourteen studies by Garcia *et al.* (2008), Alzheimer's disease was associated with chronic occupational EMR exposure.

One of the difficulties with assessing the data on EMR effects is the sheer volume of studies of different types that has been published over the past twenty years. The breadth of variances between the studies of plants, animals, and human response to various degrees of radiation is substantial. Because of this huge base of studies, most researchers have been forced to rely upon various reviews by publications and government agencies to assess the implications of this large base of varying research. These groups have assessed and compared studies to figure out whether there is a correlation between study results, and whether they are significant. Government-sponsored reviews have included the United Kingdom's National Radiological Protection Board, the Associated Universities of Oak Ridge, the French National Institute of Health and Medical Research; councils in Denmark, Sweden, Australia and Canada together with U.S. agencies such as the Environmental Protection Agency and the Department of Transportation. In addition, the U.S. National Council on Radiation Protection and Measurements and the US National Academy of Sciences have also put together major reports on EMR research.

A number of respected journals have published reviews of EMR research as well. While some of these studies have found some epidemiological evidence notable, few found conclusive results, and some have presented skeptical views of any significant positive pathological correlation with non-ionizing EMR exposure. Multiple reviews were also presented (Savitz 1993) in *Environmental Health Perspectives*. No interaction mechanism between power line EMRs and biological organisms was determined.

An electrical field is a substantially different magnetic field. An electrical field is generated when there is a charge differential between two terminating points, regardless of whether current runs between them. An electric light bulb will still generate an electric field even when it is turned off. This electrical field allows alternating current to run between the two points when the switch is eventually turned on.

A magnetic field is created by a current flowing with electricity. The magnetic field will be emitted outward with perpendicular orientation to the electrical field. However, because magnetic fields have a particular polarity or direction, a current flowing in the opposite direction placed next to the current wire will cancel the magnetic field. Most power cords with double wires (hot and ground for a circuit loop) effectively cancel the magnetic field of the incoming current directly related to the distance between the wires. An increase in this separation increases the strength of the magnetic field. This occurs in power lines, where conductors are typically separated by poles and shields for fire protection.

For these reasons, excessive magnetic fields are considered to have the greatest potential for harm. The level of potential harm is related directly to the distance from the generating source, the distance between other conductors, the size of the coils on the transformer (if any) and of course the amount of current flowing through the system. It is generally accepted that the relative magnetic field strength halves with the amount of distance from the line. In other words, a line 100-feet away will have one-quarter of the magnetic field strength of a line 50-feet away.

Li *et al.* (1997), after testing 407 residences in northern Taiwan ranging from 50 meters to 150 meters from high-voltage power lines, found that the magnetic fields at the houses ranged from .93 mG for 50 meters to between .51 and .55 milliGauss for residences under 149 meters, and .29 mG for residences beyond 149 meters.

This data is somewhat contradicted by a 1993 cohort study from the Netherlands that revealed magnetic field intensities, ranging from 1 to 11 milliGauss from two kilovolt power lines connecting to one transformer substation (Schreiber 1993).

Higher voltage wires are typically thought to be an issue because the voltage and speed is boosted to travel longer distances. With a high-speed voltage line comes an increase in magnetic field. Magnetic fields have been connected with decreased melatonin secretion

(Brainard *et al.* 1999). A number of studies have linked lower mela-tonin levels with higher incidence of a number of types of cancers. It would thus seem probable that since lower melatonin levels are associated with higher voltage, high-speed power lines could well be a mechanism for cancer (Ravindra 2006).

In comparison, a typical house or office will range from .8 to 1 mG in magnetic fields. The magnetic field strength from a kitchen appliance at close range for a person working in the kitchen is sig-nificantly greater than the strength coming from power lines 50-100 feet away. Stepping a few feet away from a microwave oven will dramatically reduce this field strength, while that same relative power line reduction will require a more significant change. A typi-cal microwave oven might cause a field strength of 1000 mG, which can be reduced to a minimal 1 mG by stepping a few feet away. Moving ones house further away from a power line obviously re-quires a significant commitment to the reduction of magnetic field strength, and a few feet will not make a significant difference.

Epidemiological studies involving electrical appliances have been limited. They are more difficult because of the control pa-rameters. Nonetheless, a few appliances have undergone controlled studies over the years. Electric blankets have undergone several studies. Some of these illustrated significantly increased risk factors for postmenopausal cancer (Vena *et al.* 1991), testicular cancer (Ver-reault 1990), and congenital defects (Dlugosz 1992).

Radio Waves

Radiofrequency waves range from about 3 hertz to 300 giga-hertz. This means their waves travel from speeds of 3 cycles per second up to 3,000,000 cycles per second. *Extremely low frequency* (ELF=3-30 Hz) and *super low frequency* (SLF=30-300 Hz) broadcast-ing has primarily been used for submarine communications, as these wavelengths transmit well through the water. This is also the fre-quency range that sound waves travel. *Ultra low frequency* (ULF=300-3000 Hz) has primarily been used in mines, where the waves can penetrate the depths. Above these levels, *very low frequency* and *low frequency* (VLF and LF = 3-300 kHz) have been used by beacons, heart rate monitors, navigation and time signaling. *Medium frequency* (300-3000 kHz) radiowaves are typically used for AM broadcasts, while *high frequency* (HF = 3-30 MHz) is used primarily for short-wave and amateur radio broadcasting. *Very high frequency* (VHF = 30-300 MHz) waves are used for FM radio, television and aircraft communications while *ultra high frequency* (UHF = 300-3000 MHz) waves are used for certain television ranges, but also cell phones, wireless LAN, GPS, Bluetooth and many two-way radios. While often considered outside the radio spectrum, *super high frequency* (SHF = 3-30 GHz) waves are used in microwave devices, some LAN wireless systems and radar. *Extremely high frequency* (EHF = 30-300 GHz) is used for long-range systems such as microwave radio and astronomy radio systems. The audio frequencies are primarily ELF through VLF brands, covering 20-20,000 Hz.

Note that EMR wavelengths inversely vary to their frequency. For naturally occurring EMR such as sunlight, the frequency will equal the speed of light divided by the wavelength. Thus, an ULF wave can range from 10,000 and 100,000 kilometers long. An UHF wave will range from one meter to ten millimeters in length, while an ELF wavelength will range from one millimeter and ten millimeters long.

Adulterated radiofrequencies have been utilized by humans for only about the last seventy-five years. Early use was primarily for radio transmission, while during the past few decades, various communication and signaling systems have been developed that utilize radiofrequencies. Radiofrequencies are generated with alternating current fed through an antenna at particular speeds and wavelengths.

Studies on radiofrequency radiation proximity at work have also studied possible reproductive and cardiovascular effects. While many of the reports are inconclusive, there have been positive correlations between radiofrequency exposure and delayed conception (Larsen *et al.* 1991), spontaneous abortion (Quellet-Hellstrom and Steward 1993; Taskinen *et al.* 1990), stillbirth (Larsen *et al.* 1991), preterm birth after father exposure (Larsen *et al.* 1991), and birth defects (Larson 1991). However, many of these results have either not been replicated or remain uncorroborated. Three studies examined male military personnel exposure to microwaves and radar (Hjollund *et al.* 1997; Lancranjan *et al.* 1975; Weyandt *et al.* 1996). All three found reductions in sperm density.

A number of animal studies have illustrated adverse health effects from radiowaves but doubt has been raised regarding the dose comparison with humans. In one study, GSM phone frequency radiowaves caused the cell death of about 2% of rat brains. Researchers hypothesized that the blood-brain barrier was being penetrated by the radiation (Salford 2003). This was correlated by three earlier studies that reported blood-brain barrier penetration with radiowave exposure (Shivers *et al.* 1987; Prato *et al.* 1990; Schirmacher *et al.* 2000). For several years following the release of this last study, other studies could not replicate the findings, nor could they establish a confirmation of the permeation of the blood-brain-barrier from radiofrequencies (Kuribayashi 2005; others). However, Shivers and colleagues, and Prato and associates had previously determined the effect of magnetic resonance imaging upon the rat brain. They showed that the exposure to radiofrequencies combined with pulsed and static magnetic fields gave rise to a significant pinocytotic transport of albumin from the capillaries into the brain.

Rates of breast cancer, endometrial cancer, testicular cancer and lung cancer have been studied with close range radiofrequency radiation, primarily in occupational settings. Slightly positive correlations with endometrial cancer (Cantor *et al.* 1995) and male breast cancer (Demers *et al.* 1991) were found. A potential link between testicular cancer and radiofrequency radiation from traffic radar guns, particularly among a small group of police officers (Davis and Mostofi 1993) was also established. Slightly increased ocular melanoma was established among occupational radiofrequency exposure (Holly *et al.* 1996) in another small group. French and Canadian utility workers were found to have an increased likelihood of lung cancer (Armstrong *et al.* 1994).

Cell phone tower radiofrequencies are popular concerns. The first cell phones communicated with analog frequencies of 450 or 900 megahertz, for example. By the 1990s, cell phones were using 1800 megahertz, and various modulation systems. Now the Universal Mobile Telecommunication System is adhered to, which uses 1900 to 2200 megahertz.

In 2000, over 80,000 cell tower base stations were in use in the United States. By 2006, this number was estimated at 175,000.

CTIA, the International Association for Wireless Telecommunications Industry, estimates that by 2010 there will be about 260,000 towers. These base stations transmit radiowaves using around 100 watts of power. The range of GSM towers is about 40 kilometers, while the CDMA and iDEN technologies offer ranges of 50 to 70 kilometers. This obviously is relative to terrain. In a hilly area, the range can be a few kilometers.

In populated areas, cell base towers are placed from one to two miles apart, while in urban areas they can be as close together as a quarter of a mile. Some cell phone bases are mounted on primary towers, and some are built onto elevated structures such as buildings and hillsides.

A base cell tower antenna is comprised of a transmitter(s), a receiver(s) – often called transceivers – an electrical power source, and various digital signal processors. The circuits will utilize copper, fiber, or microwave connections. They may be connected to the network via T1, E1, T3 and/or Ethernet connections. They are typically strung together through base station controllers and radio network controllers, typically connected to a switched telephone network system. The radio network controller will connect to the SGSN network.

There has been scant research on the risks of radiofrequency waves from radio stations or television stations. The primary reason for this appears to be that most of these have been located outside of densely populated areas, on high towers enabling greater ranges. Cell towers have created more concern because of their close proximity and relatively lower heights.

Research has suggested that exposure from cell towers is reduced by a factor of one to one hundred times inside of a building, depending upon the building materials and style of the building. However, exposure also increases with height. Upper floors can have substantially greater exposure levels than lower floors (Schuz and Mann 2000). Whether this is a factor of pure height or whether the earth provides a buffering factor is not known.

Exposure levels in regions surrounding cell towers will range from .01 to .1% of ISNIRP (International Commission on Non-Ionizing Radiation Protection) permitted levels for general public exposure directly around the station, to .1 to 1% of ISNIRP permitted levels between 100 meters and 200 meters from the tower. Beyond the 200-meter level, the exposure returns to the .01 to .1% level and reduces as the range increases. It should be noted also that exposure levels from cell phone towers are not substantially greater than exposure levels of radiofrequencies (RF) emitted by radio broadcasting towers. In one Australian study, the greatest level found was .2% (Henderson 2006).

In a 2006 randomized double-blind study performed at the Institute of Pharmacology and Toxicology at the University of Zurich (Regel *et al.*) in Switzerland, UMTS signals approximating the strength of a cell phone tower emission were tested on 117 healthy human subjects, 33 of which reported themselves as sensitive to cell towers and 84 as non-sensitive. Physiological analyses included organ-specific tests, cognitive tests, and well-being questionnaires. Apparently, significant negative physiological or cognitive results were not found, although there appeared to be a marginal effect on one of the cognitive tests for each of the two groups. Because the difference was slight, and each group (sensitive versus control) had different results, this effect was considered insignificant.

In 2006, the British medical journal (Rubin *et al.*) reported a study done at the King's College in London, which tested 60 self-reported sensitive people and 60 control subjects with no reported sensitivities. Six different symptoms such as headaches were tracked, and subjects took questionnaires in an attempt to find whether the sensitive subjects could successfully judge whether a cell tower signal was on or off. While 60% of the sensitive subjects believed the tower signals were on when they were on, 63% believed the tower signals to be on when they were indeed off.

There have also been several international studies done on radiofrequency transmissions from masts. Tests in the United States, Britain, Australia and the Vatican City have shown no or low correlation between RF levels and health effects, rendering these studies for the most part, inconclusive. One study in the Netherlands using simulated mobile phone base station transmissions did conclude, however, that the UMTS-like spectrum of cell transmission might have an adverse affect upon the well-being of questionnaire respondents.

In July of 2007, an independent team of researchers (Eltiti *et al.*) from the University of Essex reported findings from a three-year double-blind study using a special laboratory to test potential cell phone tower effects. The study included 44 people who reported sensitivity to cell phone towers and 114 healthy people who had not. The study measured various physiological factors like skin conductance, blood pressure and heart rate while being exposed (or not) to 3G tower signals. During periods where the researcher and the subject knew the signals were on, sensitive people reported feeling worse, and their physiological factors were affected negatively. However when neither the subjects nor the researchers knew the cell tower signals were on during a series of tests, there was no difference between either the sensitive or non-sensitive subjects with regard to physiological factors. In fact, only two of the forty-four sensitive subjects were able to guess the cell tower signals being on correctly while five of the control subjects (non-sensitive) were able to guess correctly. Subjects who reported sensitivities to cell phone towers prior to the study reported negative symptoms more often, regardless of whether the cell tower transmitters were on or off.

Remote and Cell Phones

Typically, a digital cell phone operates at a power range of about .25 watts, while the newest digital phones might transmit as low as .09 watts. Analog phones were much higher power transmitters. The exposure level of a cell phone will depend greatly upon the way the phone is designed. The location of the antenna and the power supply/battery will typically govern the strength of the transmission to the dermal layers of the skin. The further away the antenna is from dermal contact (hand or ear), the less exposure.

The orientation of the power supply will also govern exposure. Some phones have shielding between the power supply and the antenna and earpiece. This is thought to reduce dermal exposure. In other words, the manner of carrying and holding the phone will vary the exposure.

There is another factor called *adaptive power*. When a cell phone is further away from a tower, or in a moving car, it will typically increase its internal transceiver power to send and receive signals. This increases the level of electromagnetic exposure as the phone is boosting power and transmissions. EMR cell phone exposure is thus typically less outdoors than indoors, because there is less interference from building materials outdoors. In addition, exposure to radiowaves is greatest on the side of the head the phone is most used and closest to where the antenna is located (Dimbylow and Mann 1994).

Radiofrequencies from handset use have been confirmed to heat the ear canal. In one controlled study of 30 individuals, 900 MHz and 1800 MHz phones against the ear for more than 35 minutes resulted in an increase of 1.2-1.3 degrees F (Tahvanainen *et al.* 2007). Other studies have confirmed this effect. For this reason there has been a great concern regarding the potential for tumor development either in the brain or in the areas surrounding the ears – referred to as an *acoustic neurinoma*.

Adverse effects of tissue temperature rise are not clear, but it is thought that the body's thermoregulation mechanisms may create an increased immune burden on the body. Lab studies have suggested a one-centigrade temperature rise at the tissue level will have immunosuppressive effects (Goldstein *et al.* 2003).

The International Agency for Research into Cancer has sponsored studies in thirteen countries to study the line between cell phone usage and cancer. So far, Australia, Canada, Denmark, Finland, France, Germany, Israel, Italy, Japan, New Zealand, Norway, Sweden and Britain have participated. Through 2005, the research tracked 6,000 glioma and menigioma cases (brain tumors), 1000 acoustic neurinoma cases and 600 parotid gland cancers. Of these, the acoustic neurinoma results, primarily from Sweden, showed a significant link with handset use – from both cell phones and cordless phones. The German study also revealed a significant link between uveal melanoma and unspecified handset use. Other types of tumors had OR levels of around or just above 1 to 1.7 OR. The 2001 Swedish study on all brain tumors found a 2.4 OR link with ipsilateral cancer – more prevalent on the same side of primary handset use.

Again, we are faced with the fact that many of these associations are occurring at between 1 and 3 OR. A 2 or 3 level OR risk level creates questions in the minds of meta and review researchers. This should be combined with the fact that the rates of these tumors are so small among the general population (10-15 per 100,000 per year) for malignant brain tumors (Behin *et al.* 2003). Additionally, there is often a ten-year or more delay from exposure to diagnosis. This gives some researchers a myriad of reasons to question even the better correlations between cell phones and cancer.

Other researchers firmly disagree, stating that the weaker evidence is actually enhanced by the cancer diagnosis delay. Research from the Japanese nuclear victims of World War II has shown that many cancers arise ten to twenty years and more after the initial exposure. If we extrapolate this with cell phone use, we estimate that because cell phone use among the general population is still within this twenty-year period, especially for many younger adults (who were barely using cell phones five years ago). This means we should expect to see higher cancer rates among heavy cell phone users within the next five to ten years from now. Possibly this might be ameliorated somewhat by the improved cell phones being made now, with increased shielding (which begs the question; why did they increase the shielding if there was no danger?). Or not. We will see. The grand experiment with EMR rages on.

One of the more dramatic releases on cell phone use emerged in 2003 from a study conducted by Dr. Michael Klieeisen at Spain's Neuro Diagnostic Research Institute. This study revealed from a CATEEN scanner linked to a brainwave activity-imaging unit that radiowaves from cell phones could penetrate and interfere with the electrical activity of an eleven-year-old boy and a thirteen-year-old girl. Various hypotheses resulted from the release of this data. Among them, that radiowaves affect the moods, memory, and activities of children. Because brainwaves have been closely linked to moods, recollection, response time and other cognition skills, it is assumed that cell phone use has a disturbing effect upon cell phone users – particularly in children and adolescents.

In a 2004 study (Maier *et al.*), eleven volunteers' cognitive performance was tested with and without being exposed to electromagnetic fields similar to cell phones. Nine of the eleven (or 81.8%) showed reduced performance in cognitive testing following exposure.

It should be noted that there is a tremendous market resistance to the information that cell phones and remote phones could be dangerous when used consistently. The cell phone industry is now a multi-billion dollar international business. The damage undeniable evidence of a health risk would have upon this industry is nothing short of monumental. It goes without saying that this would also have a significant impact upon the human lifestyle.

This effect may be effectively illustrated by the events reported by Dr. George Carlo and Martin Schram in their 2001 book *Cell Phones: Invisible Hazards in the Wireless Age*. Dr. Carlo was a well-respected epidemiologist/research scientist and pathologist. He was retained by the cell phone industry's chief lobbyist to study and comment on research regarding potential dangers of cell phone use. However, it was not expected that Dr. Carlo would speak out against cell phone use after examining the research data. In his book, Dr. Carlo describes the extraordinary efforts of the cell phone industry to discredit him. As Dr. Carlo began to announce negative cancer-related findings, his clients began to apply both political and financial pressure upon him.

We should however note that although U.S. brain cancer rates have increased substantially over the past three decades, brain cancer incidence increased until 1987, and has been slowly decreasing from that point (Deorah *et al.* 2006). This statistic does not concur with a model of increasing brain cancer rates with increasing cell phone usage. Quite possibly, some of the environmental etiologies involved in brain cancer prior to 1987 have been somewhat mitigated. Perhaps some of the toxin exposure levels – such as the rampant use of DDT and toxic waste dumping in waterways – have been curtailed due to some of the EPA actions of the 1960s and 1970s – decreasing brain cancer rates in the years following. We also cite further controls on nuclear leaks and a massive reduction in tobacco use. Epidemiologically, these could well be masking a slow rise in brain cancer levels due to cell phone use.

Cancer is not the only issue to consider with regard to cell phones, however. Researchers have examined other disorders with respect to radiofrequency exposure. Heavy cell users commonly report a wide variety of negative symptoms. In a study of 300 individuals at Alexandria University in Egypt (Salama and Naga 2004), cell phone usage was positively correlated with complaints of headaches, earaches, sense of fatigue, sleep disturbance, concentration difficulty and burning-face sensation. The results showed that 68% of the study population used cell phones. All of the above health complaints were significantly higher among the cell phone users, and 72.5% of the cell phone users had health complaints. The frequency duration of cell phone usage was also extrapolated together with health complaints, and it was discovered that the higher the cell phone use, the greater the incidence of health complaints. While the burning-face sensation complaint correlated positively with call frequency per day, complaints of fatigue also significantly correlated (positively) with both call duration and call frequency.

The warming of the ear, face and the scalp around our ear from cell phone use is logically taking place as a result of frequency and waveform interference between our body's natural waveforms and these synthetic waveforms. Our body's natural waveforms include the shorter waves of the brain and nerves, and the weaker bio-photon waveforms of the cells, along with the molecular electro-magnetic bonding waveforms within DNA. Should electronically driven waveforms interfere with these natural biowaves, the molecular bonding structures of our genetic information could gradually become deranged.

The effects of this interference should appear on a number of fronts. We should see lower cognition levels and brain fog, as unnatural waveforms interfere with our brainwave mapping system. We should see body temperature interference within the basal cell network. We should see damage to the blood-brain barrier and damage to nerve and brain cells. These effects should release greater levels of radical species from the imbalanced molecular structures – damaging cells and tissues. All of these effects have been documented in the research.

This waveform interference mechanism is illustrated by a recent study (Thaker *et al.* 2008) showing that a certain popular brand of MP3 player will interfere with the mechanisms of a pacemaker if held close to the chest for about five seconds. Appliance interference has been directly correlated with waveform interference. This is one reason why the U.S. Federal Communications Commission closely monitors and licenses bandwidths. When we consider that the body maintains various natural biowave "bandwidths" as it cycles hormones, thermoregulation, cortisol, melatonin and the Krebs energy cycle to name a few, it is not difficult to connect the wave-form interference of cell phones and other appliances with the disruption of these natural cycles.

Video Display Terminals

VDTs and televisions emit about 60 hertz of electromagnetic fields. Although a number of early studies suggested the potential of a health risk, many studies over the past few years have suggested that VDTs pose little if any health risks. The National Academy of Sciences reviewed a number of studies in 1999 and stated, *"....the current body of evidence does not show that exposure to these fields presents a human health hazard..."* In 1994, the American Medical Association stated, *"no scientifically documented health risk has been associated with the usually occurring levels of electromagnetic fields..."* Their review included both epidemiological studies and various other direct studies of EMR effects from terminals.

Another report, published in *Lancet,* the British Medical Association's journal, documented the largest childhood study comparing childhood leukemia and cancer rates and exposure to 50-hertz non-ionizing magnetic fields. No link was found.

The National Radiological Protection Board in 1994 confirmed that while existing conditions might be aggravated, their review of the research showed no link between skin diseases or cataract formation and VDT use. However, the board's Chairman Sir Richard Doll, did confirm that VDT use might aggravate conditions that have already formed.

In addition, a bevy of clinical research regarding pregnancy outcome for those working around or on computers has failed to show any links between miscarriage or birth defects and VDT use. The National Radiological Protection Board from Oxford, U.K. confirmed this in a review of the research.

In 1998, the International Commission on Non-Ionizing Radiation Protection submitted low emission field guidelines. They suggested an upper limit of magnetic field exposure of 833 milli-Gauss (mG). The electric field limit was set at 4,167 volts per meter (V/m).

Both VDTs and televisions are far below these exposure levels when measured individually.

155

Regardless of these reports, problems associated with vision, fatigue and headaches have been reported from VDT use. These problems have been attributed to such ergonomic issues as the potential for glare on the screen, lighting location with the position of the screen, the distance from the screen, and whether there are regular breaks from looking at the screen.

Other issues reported have been associated with static electricity generated through the keyboard and screen, posture problems, and repetitive injuries such as keyboarding without rest, which can create a risk of carpal tunnel and other motor difficulties.

As for television, there have been numerous efforts to study the effects of television on children and adults. Most of these have leaned towards its behavioral effects, but a few have reported significant effects on physical health. In 2007, Crönlein et al. found a significant link between television viewing and adolescent children insomnia. Thakkar et al. (2006) and Paavonen et al. (2006) found that watching violence on television increased insomnia and sleep disturbances among young children. Bickham and Rich (2006) showed that increased television viewing – especially violent TV – was associated negatively with friendships. Hammermeister et al. (2005) showed that viewers who watched two hours or less television per day had a more positive psychosocial health profile. Viner and Cole (2005) determined that early childhood television viewing was associated with people who had a higher body mass index later in life. Other studies have also correlated increased television viewing with childhood obesity (Robinson 2001).

Meanwhile Zimmerman and Christakis (2005) found that children who watched a significant amount of television before the age of three years (2.2 hours/day) scored lower on Peabody reading comprehension, memory and intelligence testing at ages six and seven. Hancox et al. (2005) found in New Zealand that increased television viewing was associated with higher dropout rates and lower rates of university attendance. Collins et al. (2004) found that watching sex on television increases sex activity at a younger age in children. Huesmann et al. (2003) found that watching violence on television increased violent behavior during adulthood. Vallani (2001) illustrated that research since 1990 progressively showed that increased television viewing increases violent behavior, aggression, and high-risk behavior such as smoking, drinking, and promiscuousness.

However, Anderson *et al.* (2001) indicated that television content might have more to do with these associations. 570 adolescents were studied from preschool, and their programming was monitored. Educational program watching was linked to higher grades, increased reading, greater creativity and fewer violent activities.

Microwaves

Microwave ovens produce two different forms of radiation: High frequency radiowaves produce electromagnetic frequencies in the range of 2450 megahertz and magnetic fields at 60 hertz. The central question is whether this is enough bombardment to cause harm to the food. While some claims have been made that microwave ovens cause the food particles to spin and rotate, this statement has not been confirmed by scientific investigation. What we know is that the microwaves increase the waveform energy states of the molecules using thin microwave beams in much the same way fire increases energy states. Whether this is accompanied by a spinning or rotation of the molecule appears to be speculative, though it appears likely – understanding the physics involved.

Indeed, microwaves do create unnatural molecular structure results. A well-cooked microwave dinner reveals dry and rubbery textures not seen in other forms of cooking. Is microwaved food healthy?

Dr. Robert Becker (1985) reported that various disorders such as cardiovascular difficulties, stress, headaches, dizziness, anxiety, irritability, insomnia, reproductive disorders, and cancer occurred in the Soviet Union among microwave-exposed workers when the Soviets were developing radar during the 1950s. In fairness, though technically correct, these were people working amongst microwave transmissions, not eating microwaved dinners.

Dr. Becker also reported that research from Russia indicated nutritional reductions of sixty to ninety percent in microwave oven tests. Decreases in bioavailable vitamin Bs, vitamin C, vitamin E, minerals, and oil nutrients were observed. Alkaloids, glucosides, galactosides and nitrilosides – all phytonutrients – were found damaged by microwaving. Some proteins were found to be denatured.

Research (Knize *et al.* 1999) at the University of California Lawrence Livermore Laboratory concluded that microwaves produced heterocyclic aromatic amines and polycyclic aromatic hydrocarbons. Both are suspected carcinogens. Frying meats also produces polycyclic aromatic hydrocarbons (Felton *et al.* 1994).

Dr. Lita Lee wrote in her 1989 book, *Microwaves and Microwave Ovens* that the Atlantis Rising Educational Center in Oregon reported that a number of carcinogens form during the microwaving of nearly all types of foods. Microwaving meats caused formation of the carcinogen d-nitrosodiethanolamine. Microwaving milk and grains converted amino acids into carcinogenic compounds. Thawing frozen fruit by microwave converted glucosides and galactosides into carcinogenic chemicals. Short-term microwaving converted alkaloids from plant foods into carcinogenic compounds. Carcinogenic free radicals formed during the microwaving of root vegetables, according to this report.

In December of 1989, the British Medical Association's *Lancet* reported that microwaves converted trans-amino acids to cis-isomers in baby formulas. Another amino acid, L-proline, converted to a d-isomer version. These isomers have been classified as neurotoxins (toxic to the nerves) and nephrotoxins (toxic to the kidneys).

Swiss food scientist Dr. Hans Ulrich Hertel and Dr. Bernard Blanc of the Swiss Federal Institute of Technology reported in a 1991 paper that microwave food created cancerous effects within the bloodstream. The small study had eight volunteers consume either raw milk; conventionally cooked milk, pasteurized milk; microwave-cooked milk; organic raw vegetables; conventionally-cooked vegetables; the same vegetables frozen and warmed in a microwave; or the same vegetables cooked in the microwave oven. Blood tests were taken before and after eating. Subjects who ate microwaved milk or vegetables had decreased hemoglobin levels, increased cholesterol levels and decreased lymphocyte levels. The increase in leucocytes concerned Dr. Hertel the most. Increased leukocyte levels in the bloodstream are generally connected with infection or tissue damage.

The controls in some of these studies may be in question, however. For example, in Dr. Hertel's study he was a participant, the group knew whether the food was microwaved or not, and the group members were predominantly macrobiotic. The Russian studies and the *Atlantis Rising* report statistics all come unconfirmed from secondary sources.

Various forms of cooking will also destroy nutrients and generate carcinogens – especially frying and barbequing. Overcooking in general destroys nutrients and can create a variety of free radicals that can be tumor forming if eaten in excess.

There are other dangers reported from microwaves. The leakage of various toxins from packaging during microwaving has been documented. A 1990 *Nutrition Action Newsletter* reported that various toxins will leach onto microwaved foods from food containers. Suspected carcinogens including benzene, toluene and xylene were among chemicals released into food. Also found was polyethylene terphtalate (PET). Various plasticizers are almost certainly to be included in this list, as they will quite easily outgas when heated.

In addition, microwaving – -unless done for extended periods – rarely completely sterilizes a food. This should be a warning for all those who pack leftovers into storage containers and assume a few minutes in the microwave will produce a sterile, cooked food. This fact has become obvious from the *Salmonella* outbreaks among those who took food home in doggie bags to microwave later.

Approaching this logically, it is apparent that nature did not design food to be cooked in microwaves.

This is evidenced by a simple experiment conducted in 2006. Marshall Dudley's granddaughter completed a Knoxville science fair project that compared plant water feeding between stove-boiled filtered water and the same filtered water source microwaved. She started with sets of plants of identical species, age, and health. One of each set was fed filtered water boiled in a pan and cooled. She fed another the same filtered water, but microwaved until boiling and cooled. This 'watering study' went on for a period of nine days, and pictures of the plant sets (which sat together in identical potted condition) were taken each day.

The simple assessment of each plant's health was clear by looking at the photographs. Each day the plant watered with microwaved-water looked worse. It became increasingly withered and slumped over in obvious stress. By the ninth day, the microwave-watered plant had lost most of its leaves. Meanwhile, the boiled-watered plant stood tall with crisp green leaves, growing healthier by the day.

Radon

As research in the nineties focused on power lines, research has illuminated the fact that electromagnetic fields can interact with various elements in the atmosphere, creating radon gas. A further potential danger has been proposed for households not properly wired with copper and insulation. A lack of shielding can also increase the potential interaction of household electricity with radon.

Radon 222 comes primarily from the nuclear decay of uranium. This natural process takes place within the earth. As this decay proceeds, radon gas is released, together with decay byproducts, called *radon daughters* or *radon progeny*. These particles are known carcinogens. Should we breathe these particles, they can be caught in the lungs. Breathing radon gas delivers the potential of it continuing to decay inside our bodies. This will effectively deposit the radioactive daughters inside our bodies.

The National Council on Radiation Protection and Measurement has developed a maximum safe dosage of radon to be 200 mrem per year.

The relationship between radon and outdoor power lines has not been clearly established, because in order to measure the interaction, an aerosol component (a pollutant of some sort) must accompany the electromagnetic field. Nonetheless, significant *radon daughters* have been measured (Henshaw *et al.* 1998) among power line fields.

The subsequent dose and tolerance of radon particles in the human body is also in question. In some research, heavy electromagnetic fields have been shown to penetrate with no more than about .0001 of the original field strength of radon emissions. Still this penetration effect alerted researchers to the fact that there might be a radon penetration into the lungs and basal tissues of the body (Fews *et al.* 1999).

The link between radon and lung cancer has become more evident in recent research. Lung cancer has been the most prevalent form of cancer worldwide since 1985, and has been responsible for more than one million deaths worldwide. The highest rates of lung cancer occurred in 2002 in North America and Northern or Eastern Europe. Although smoking is widely considered to be the primary etiology of lung cancer, uranium miners – who are exposed to increased levels of radon along with dust – experience higher rates of lung cancer (Tomasek *et al.* 2008). Epidemiological studies on radon-exposure and miners have also revealed that thousands of miners die per year of radon exposure (Field *et al.* 2006).

Research has illustrated that while living outdoors does not increase ones risk of lung cancer, unnatural living or working quarters without enough ventilation can lead to a drawing in and encapsulation of radon radiation. A household with poor ventilation poses a higher risk of radon exposure than a well-ventilated house. This is exasperated by other electromagnetic radiation in the local environment. Research has illustrated that ventilation around electromagnetic current exposure is an absolute requirement because of a release of radon daughters into the immediate atmosphere (Karpin 2005).

Darby *et al.* (2005) reported in the *British Medical Journal* on a collaborative analysis of thirteen case studies of 7,148 lung cancer cases together with 14,208 control subjects. This found that increased radon exposure is responsible for about 2% of European cancer deaths. Further research has revealed that most buildings, especially work environments that are full of various power lines and equipment, retain higher levels of radon. Radon levels are additionally increased with unventilated soils, higher air temperatures and higher atmospheric levels. Higher household radon levels are particularly associated with leaking and unventilated soils in the house. This research has caused legislation in many states in the U.S. requiring property sellers to disclose known radon issues.

The majority of our everyday radiation input comes from radon. Natural concentrations of radon are found in some granites, limestones and sandstones. Higher radon levels come from disturbed ground. Disturbing the normal landscape allows more permeability, allowing the release of the normally contained daughters. Once a house is built upon disturbed ground, the radon can come in through cracked foundations and spaces around piping and wiring. Because radon gas is pulled in through pressure changes within the house created by temperature gradients, it is important that our houses be well ventilated. This is particularly significant during the nighttime and during cold weather, as the warmer temperatures inside with colder temperatures outside cause the most pressure differential – the *Bernoulli effect*. Ventilation will not only allow the escape of indoor radon gas, but it will release some of this pressure, resulting in a lower draw of radon gas into the house.

Household radon levels tend to increase dramatically during the winter, and decrease substantially during the summer for these reasons. Radon levels also go up dramatically during the nighttime hours, as the outdoor temperature cools. This is when ventilation is most important.

Disturbed landscaping ground can also leak increased radon daughters.

Magnetic Anomaly

Nature's magnetic fields surround us, and pose little threat. Many species utilize nature's magnetic fields to navigate migration and nesting. In other words, our cells are tuned to the geomagnetic fields of the sun and the earth.

Synthetic magnetic fields, on the other hand, are dispersed with the distribution of unnatural alternating current. The proliferation of electricity and electrical appliances created by power-generating plants that convert nature's kinetic energy into alternating current has deluged our atmosphere with unnatural magnetism.

Most early research on the health effects of electrical appliances and wires focused on the electrical fields and ignored the magnetic fields given off by appliances. While most electrical fields are shielded by insulators within most appliances, magnetic fields can be more disruptive and insidious to the health of the body. This is because they can directly interfere with the body's internal biowaves. Normally, synchronic and harmonic biowaves – including brainwaves, nerve firings, and so on – travel with synchronicity throughout the body.

A magnetic field surrounding the body can induce an abnormal electrical current flow within the body. In a Swedish study (Wilen *et al.* 2004) of RF operators exposed to high levels of magnetic fields, currents were induced within the body at mean levels of 101 mA and maximum levels of one Amp. During this study, exposure levels correlated positively with the prevalence of fatigue, headaches, warm sensations in the hands, slower heart rates and more brady-cardia episodes among the subjects.

In a study done by the Fred Hutchinson Cancer Research Center and the Epidemiology Division of Public Health Services in Seattle, Washington (Davis *et al.* 2001), 203 women aging from 20-74 years with no breast cancer history were studied between 1994 and 1996. Magnetic field and ambient light in the bedroom were measured for a 72-hour period during two seasons of the year. Urine samples were taken on three consecutive nights for each subject. After adjusting for hours of daylight, older age, higher body mass, alcohol use and medication use, those women with higher bedroom levels of magnetic fields had lower concentrations of 6-sulfatoxy-melatonin. It was thus concluded that increased levels of synthetic magnetic fields depress nocturnal melatonin.

While this illustrates how unnatural magnetism can significantly affect the body's biochemical rhythms, reduced melatonin also causes negative effects throughout the body. Over several decades since melatonin was discovered in 1958 by Dr. Aaron Lerner and his Yale colleagues, decreased melatonin levels have been linked to a variety of pathologies and immune function deficiencies.

A three milliGauss magnetic field at 60 Hertz will induce about one-billionth amp per square centimeter of the body. A magnetic field at 120 Hz frequency will have double the current effect the same field will have at 60 Hz. A typical American office building or home – filled with various electrical appliances – will contain magnetic fields at levels between .8 and 1 milliGauss. In a study done at a Canadian school by Akbar-Khanzadeh in 2000, workers, school-teachers and administrative staff environments had magnetic field exposure levels ranging from .2 to 7.1 mG.

MilliGauss levels will be substantially higher in instrument-heavy environments. Hood *et al.* (2000) recorded the pilot's cockpits of a Boeing 767 with magnetic field levels of 6.7 milliGauss, while the Boeing 737 recorded at 12.7 mG of magnetic field strength. Nicholas *et al.* (1998) documented a mean magnetic field strength of 17 mG among the cockpits of B737, B757, DC9 and L1011 planes. Meanwhile, cabin measurements ranged from a high of 8 mG in the forward serving areas to 6 mG in the first class seats and 3 mG in the economy seats.

Rail maintenance workers experience magnetic field levels from 3 to 18 mG (Wenzl 1997). In a study published in the *Journal of the Canadian Dental Association* (Bohay *et al.* 1994), dental operating rooms with various ultrasonic scalars, amalgamators, and x-ray equipment revealed magnetic fields ranging from 1.2 to 2225 mG, with equipment distances from zero to thirty centimeters.

Most of these magnetic field readings were accompanied by lower level radiation frequencies ranging from 25 hertz to 100 hertz (though the airline cockpits research recorded up to 800 hertz).

In a population study of 969 women in San Francisco, miscarriage levels positively correlated with higher magnetic field exposure. Li *et al.* (2002) concluded that fields in the region of 16 mG or higher produced the greatest risk of miscarriage. While higher levels of magnetic fields have been shown not to significantly affect nervous system biowaves such as cardiac pacemakers (Graham *et al.* 2000), 12 milliGauss magnetic fields operating from radiation frequencies of 60 hertz were shown to block the inhibition of human breast cancer cells by both melatonin and tamoxifen *in vitro*. While melatonin and tamoxifen have different mechanisms of retarding cancer growth, it was confirmed by Harland and Liburdy (1997) that synthetic magnetic fields prevented their immunity effects. When we consider that the magnetic fields blocked the immune activities of *both* biochemicals – which work within different mechanisms – the affect of synthetic magnetic fields on the human body illustrates an *immune system magnetic interference* model.

This magnetic field interference model of electromagnetic exposure is further supported by research published in 2002 by Saunders and Jefferys. Brain tissue testing showed that even very low frequency electric and weak magnetic field exposure will induce electric fields and currents inside the body. These fields excited various nerve cells and retinal cells, inducing abnormal metabolic activity.

The immune system magnetic interference model mechanism is further confirmed by a study of magnetic and electric fields on neural cells by Blackman (1993). While magnetic fields stimulated abnormal neurite outgrowth between 22 and 40 mG, increased electric fields did not stimulate the same morphological change.

In contrast, the natural magnetic field strength of the earth ranges from about .2 gauss to .6 gauss (200-600 mG) – often also measured as .05 Tesla (1 Tesla=10,000 gauss). To give some reference with nature's levels, an MRI magnet will range from one to three Tesla, or 10,000 to 30,000 gauss. This is equivalent to 10,000,000-30,000,000 mG.

We should also note that the earth and sun's natural magnetic fields resonate with living organisms. The earth's magnetic field direction maintains a consistent rhythmicity, shifting slowly over time. The sun's biomagnetism is also rhythmic, as solar storm activity has illustrated. The combination of these two natural forms of natural magnetism resonates with the polarity of our cells. In comparison, our synthetic alternating electromagnetism interferes destructively with these natural forms of radiation. How do we know this? We can see the physiological effects of this interference. We can see the heating of the body as the cell phone research discussed earlier. We can see the increased fatigue, mood and cognition changes from the studies quoted earlier. We can see the increased occurrences of different types of cancers – as studies discussed earlier revealed among larger population groups. This research together illustrates that the natural EMR earthly organisms have been exposed to for millions of years resonates with our physiology and metabolism, while these new forms conflict – in one respect or another – with our bodies.

Strategies for Combating Unhealthy EMR

* **Proximity and tolerance:** How much EMR we can tolerate depends upon the type of EMR, its proximity, and the strength of our body's defense systems. These effects were studied intensely during the 1940s, as the U.S. military measured the effects of nuclear explosions with respect to proximity.

* **Ionizing or non-ionizing?** We should determine whether the EMR source is emitting ionizing or non-ionizing radiation. Many appliance manuals give the emission levels.

Other sources can be found on the internet. Ionizing radiation should be avoided or minimized to the greatest degree possible.

* **Power lines:** We might consider selecting housing that is at least 100 feet away from any high-frequency power line, and further for a large transformer. Certainly, this should be the case when having a baby or young child in the house.

* **Surge Protectors:** Running our power cords through surge protectors and switching them off after using the appliance is a good idea. This can reduce the amount of idling power moving through the appliance. This can also lower electric bills and reduce house, power line and grid loads.

* **Cell use:** We can limit our cell phone use to urgent or important calls, talk briefly, and use a headset or better yet the cell phone's speaker. Bluetooth headsets emit 2.4 GHz short-range radiofrequencies. Though non-ionizing, there is little research on the long-term effects of this technology. Wires can have their own effects, although a shielded, double-strand wire will emit little in the way of magnetic fields.

* **Measure:** A TriField® EMR meter can be used to measure our workplace, home, phone, vehicle and other environment. We can use this to determine our safe zones. Depending upon our sensitivity, magnetic field levels over 5-6 mG cause concern, especially for any length of time.

* **Assess:** We can also judge whether our EMR dose might be burdensome by assessing how we are feeling when we use these devices. Do we feel dizzy? Tired? Do we have brain fog? Does part of our body feel hot or feverish? These symptoms can lead to more serious health concerns later.

* **Field canceling equipment:** There are a number of field canceling devices on the market. While lead and nickel aprons and garments have been shown to protect against EMR doses in clinical settings, the effects of biowave products on the market are controversial, and beyond the scope of this discussion. Some, however, present studies to back

up their value. They might well be considered for those in heightened EMR environments or those with sensitivities.

* **Scans:** Lead aprons should always be worn whenever taking x-rays. CAT-scans can be questioned and avoided if unnecessary.

* **Tanning beds:** The decision on whether to sunbathe using a tanning bed should be made based not just on the UV levels. It should also be tested for magnetic dose and other radiation. See page 209. Consider the natural alternative.

* **Contact:** Contact with EMR appliances should be as brief as possible. We can turn the knob or dial then step away. At three feet, EMR from most electric appliances falls off rapidly. For televisions, this expands to about ten feet due to cathode ray screen magnetism. We can keep a distance of at least five feet away from a working microwave oven. Laptops should be taken off our laps whenever possible. Hands and wrists should be kept off the surface as much as possible. A peripheral keyboard should be considered.

* **Biowave strength:** The stronger our body's internal waveform resonance is, the more we will be able to resist the negative effects of the synthetic EMR of our environment.

* **Solar biowave strength:** The radiation from the sun can significantly strengthen the body's resonance of nature's rhythms and internal metabolism. When our body absorbs the sun's rays, our own waves begin to resonate with the sun's radiation. This can be compared to striking a chord or tuning fork in a room full of instruments tuned to the same key. As the sound vibrates through the standing instruments, the chord begins to resonate through those instruments, because they are tuned to the same frequency due to their structure (i.e., string tautness and chamber). Thus the other instruments begin to resonate can vibrate at the same frequency at an increased volume. This can also be seen with two tuning forks of the same key. As one is struck, the other begins to vibrate. Just being in the sun for

a minimum of 20-30 minutes every day or after EMR exposure can reset and significantly retrain the body's biowaves.

* **Resonate:** The sun's waveforms resonate with the earth, moon, stars, oceans, rivers, colors, plants and so many elements within nature. After millions of years of entrainment, the human organism is tuned into these same waves. Connecting with these elements will also help retrain our body's internal waves and rhythms. A daily course of outdoor exercise, whole foods, fresh water and quality sleep will support this strategy, reducing the body's stressload caused by an environment of artificial electromagnetic radiation.

Chapter Six

The Colors of Health

It was 1666 when Sir Isaac Newton first projected the sun's rays onto a wall after passing them through a prism and a narrow slit. As he contemplated the amazing rainbow of colors on the wall, he considered the cause. Did these come from the light or the prism? Rene Descartes had tried to explain it as refracted light – the colors were created by the refraction angle. Newton provided the answer to this debate as he then passed the light coming from one prism through another prism, which changed the color rays back to the original single white ray. Upon passing through yet a third prism, the light again resumed the color spectrum. This clarified to Newton that the refraction explanation could not provide the solution. If so, the second prism would yield yet more colors rather than reverting back to white light. Light, Newton proposed, must actually contain these colors. The concept of the *electromagnetic spectrum* was born.

Current instrumentation indicates that the visible spectrum is composed of red, orange, yellow, green, blue, violet, and ultra violet waveforms. Each of these waveforms has a distinctive wavelength and frequency, which gives it a unique perception of color. The rate of oscillation is different between each color. In essence, each color beats to its own drum. The smallest wavelengths of light have been observed to have the highest energy potentials. Violet for example, has a wavelength of about 375-450 nanometers. Red has one of the longer wavelengths, at 625-750 nanometers.

When color radiation strength is measured, violet has the potential to create more energetic change than the red part of the spectrum. Thus, we can say that its wavelength is inversely relative to its energy potential. This relationship between the various color wavelengths and their ability to affect distinct electron energy orbitals indicates a waveform relationship between colors and the periodic table.

Sir Newton proposed the spectrum of color could be arranged within a circle, with each color relating to a particular musical note and planet within the solar system. Although he missed several planets we now recognize – and his red range failed to reveal purple as it ranges to black – the color-harmonic concept certainly made sense to Sir Newton and his colleagues. As we broaden our view of the color spectrum with our awareness of polarity, we can reconsider this cyclical view. While light's alternating magnetic and electrical properties seem to make it impervious to the effects of the earth's magnetism, color is perceived when light interacts with the elements in our atmosphere. Rainbows are a good example of this. As light refracts through water vapor, displays of majestically brilliant color result. The aurora borealis also illustrates interactive effect between solar influence and atmospheric elements, as solar storm waveforms are trapped within the magnetosphere of the earth. As the energy levels of these atmospheric particles become excited, fantastic shapes and colors are seen in the skies.

The confluence of spectra in the electromagnetic is codified as light. Light in turn is captured within the umbrella of an all-encompassing *white light*. The white light has never been visually proven to exist, although Georg Cantor, a German mathematician at the turn of the nineteenth century and inventor of the *set theory*, spent many years attempting to prove the *continuum hypothesis*. The continuum hypothesis related finite sets to infinite sets. Extended into the plane of spectra, this continuum would connect visible light to an all-encompassing white light.

The white light, first documented in the ancient *Vedas* of India, has been discussed for thousands of years. Here the white light is referred to as the *Brahman effulgence* – the emanation from the Supreme Being. This effulgence is considered by the *Vedas* to be the source of the physical universe. The white light has since been documented in many other texts as a vehicle for transcendence.

The concept of the white light containing many other spectra of material densities and waveforms is quite similar to the notion of visible light rays containing the various spectra, visible as colors as they refract and reflect through our environment.

Color, or *chromatics,* is the translation of particular energy waveforms by the photoreceptor neurons (primarily the cones) of the eyes. This means that colors have a number of characteristics besides what our minds perceive as color. William Snow, M.D. documented that blind people can perceive color without the use of eyesight. He explained that the *"radiant light, heat and color are capable of setting up responsive vibrations in animal tissue, inducing responses relative to their intensity.... their wavelengths and frequencies."*

We have discovered through research that other rays of the electromagnetic spectrum are capable of unique physical effects. Consider cosmic rays and gamma rays, which can penetrate tissue, causing various organ and cell damage. Consider x-rays, with their potential for radiation damage with too much exposure. Consider ultraviolet rays with their potential to damage or mutate skin cells. Consider radio and television waves with the ability to carry information through buildings and other physical obstructions. The visible spectrum contains waveforms within the same range of spectra. The colors of the visible spectrum certainly influence physical structure just as do these other waveforms. However, their effects are generally more subtle and less damaging. Similarly, each color has distinct effects.

Color and light is required for long-term health and disease prevention. Research has illustrated that when a person is entrained to an indoor darkened habitat, the risk of depression grows substantially. Along with depression comes the risk of various other diseases such as fibromyalgia, back pain, digestive difficulties, decreased circulation and so on. While some research links these disorders to the body not getting enough vitamin D, others link these to the suppression of melatonin, serotonin and dopamine. Still others have associated these disorders with simply not having enough of nature's colors. We would suggest that perhaps all of the above are applicable.

Color has been used therapeutically for thousands of years with overwhelming success. It has been an important element of Ayurvedic, Chinese and Egyptian medicinal therapies. Goethe's 1810 book, *Theory of Colours* related color with Hippocratic medicine. He described the four basic colors intertwining with the four basic humours of the physical body within a circular wheel, which he coined the *"Temperamental Rose."* Goethe tested subjects and moods, describing character associations with colors, stating that, *"Every colour produces a corresponding influence on the mind."* Light and color therapy has been used amongst psychologists thereafter. Colors were used therapeutically in European asylums. Painted walls with violet or blue brought about a calming effect for anxious patients; while red, yellow and orange brought about increased activity among depressed patients.

The Ayurvedic science utilized color therapy using gems for thousands of years. Utilizing some of these principles, during the first part of the century, an Indian Colonel and self-described metaphysician and psychologist named Dinshah Ghadiali wrote and lectured famously about color therapy. In 1920, he invented a machine called the *Spectro-Chrome*. Equipped with a 1000-watt light bulb, the device had five sliding glass color plates that could be mixed and matched to create up to twelve colors. Ghadiali's instruction manual for the device – *The Spectro-Chrome Metry Encyclopaedia* – documented various therapeutic case histories of the machine's use. While Ghadiali was subsequently dubbed a quack and his machine described as a fraud by the FDA and others in the medical establishment, some 10,000 of his devices were sold and used by a wide range of healthcare providers for many decades. There were also several other similar *chromo-therapy* devices commercialized in that era. Ghadiali's was simply one of the best known. Ghadiali was said to have been influenced by Edwin Babbitt's *The Principles of Light and Color* (1878). Babbitt's book proposed that everyone has a distinct energy color. Babbit suggested illness is at least partially caused by disturbing our unique color balance. Healing, he proposed, could be hastened by re-establishing ones color balance. A schoolteacher, Mr. Babbit also invented a popular device for this purpose, called the *Chromolume*.

In 1946, Ghadiali was tried and eventually convicted of fraud. The FDA put the theory of color therapy on trial along with Ghadiali himself, and color therapy was functionally discredited in western medicine. Ironically, in that same year, a Swiss psychologist named Dr. Max Luscher designed a well-received study using colors to assess personality characteristics along with a risk assessment of potential disorder trends. Developed for psychiatrists and physicians, Luscher's color test indicated patients with higher risk factors for ailments of cardiac, cerebral, or gastro-intestinal origin, depending upon the types of colors the subject selected. His test became a standard among therapists, as it proved clinically useful.

Indeed, marketers and advertisers – who have been successfully using color in their marketing campaigns and packaging – have drawn upon a wealth of practical and measured experience relating colors with purchase decisions. It is for this reason we see fast food restaurants advertising in yellows and oranges – hunger colors. Banks, on the other hand, will pick blues and grays with some reds showing stability and professionalism. Healthy food brands will choose greens and browns to appeal to the healthy ideals of some consumers. Some marketing research has indicated that green is by far the most appealing color to food consumers. For this reason, we see lots of greens among labels on our supermarket shelves.

The use of color in the practice of psychotherapy has remained somewhat consistent over the past century despite the FDA's case against Ghadiali. Over the last two decades, controlled research has increasingly confirmed color's therapeutic effects. Today color therapy systems like *Colorpuncture* (Peter Mandel) and *Chromo-pressure* (Charles McWilliams) are emerging, combining color therapy with other established therapeutic methods (Cocilovo 1999).

There is a volume of research now confirming the usefulness of color therapies. In a study done by Lund Institute of Technology researchers (Kuuler *et al.* 2006) on 988 subjects in indoor work environments, it was concluded that brighter colors and lighting created higher moods among workers in four different countries.

In 1992, poor reading children were studied by researchers in the psychology department of the University of New Orleans (Williams *et al.*). Color overlay intervention increased reading comprehension in about 80% of the children.

Hypertension has been successfully treated with color therapy (Kniazeva *et al.* 2006). Preterm jaundiced infants have been successfully treated with blue and turquoise lighting. Significant reductions in plasma bilirubin have been achieved with color therapy (Ebbesen *et al.* 2003). The application of ultraviolet B light resulted in a lowering of blood pressure in Krause *et al.* (1998).

The visible part of the electromagnetic spectrum ranges in wavelength from 380 nanometers to 740 nanometers. Within this range, the color red has the longest wavelength, ranging from 625 to 740 nanometers. Meanwhile, orange ranges from around 590 to 625 nanometers; yellow ranges from around 565 to 590 nm; green from 500 to 565 nanometers; blue from 450 to 485; and purple from about 310 to 380 nanometers. Of course, as the wavelength increases, the speed or frequency of each waveform cycle decreases. Red ranges from a frequency of 405 to 480 terahertz (10^{12} hertz) while on the other side of the visual spectrum, purple ranges from 790 to 840 terahertz.

The color spectrum is called *continuous* because there is no cessation or absolute break between colors. Rather, the true color of a range is apparent in the middle while the edges of the color transitions into the next color, rendering a mixing of the two colors. For example, an indigo transition between purple and blue may be apparent from some observers, and cyan should appear during the green and blue transition.

Through a variant mixing of these central colors, the mind perceives thousands if not millions of colors. Some researchers have documented up to 10 million colors as potentially distinguishable by humans.

The eyes are equipped with two visual receptors: rods and cones. The cones of the eyes are the primary receptors of bright light and the color spectrum. Humans typically have three kinds of cone cells, each with a different pigment: one is sensitive to the short violet color waves; one is sensitive to the medium green waves; and one is sensitive to the longer yellow waveforms. Cones are not very sensitive to light, yet they pick up colors better in brighter light than in darker light. The rods are primarily light-sensitive cells, and thus they are useful for night vision. In fact, rods will usually only begin functioning during weaker light, distinguishing primarily black and white images.

The perception of distinct colors takes place through a contrasting process between the three types of cone cells and a *bleaching* out of others. Each different cone type has specific photoreceptors oriented to receive particular wavelengths of light. Each particular wavelength will stimulate a specific type of cone over another. A blending of multiple images from each type of cone is transmitted through the optic nerve and brain cells, providing a pallet view of various colors on the mind's screen.

The conversion of light into the neural pulses takes place through a transduction process. Like many other sensory receptors in the body, cone photoreceptor pigments become polarized by particular waveforms. When light of a particular waveform strikes a

receptor, a depolarization takes place. The depolarized photoreceptor acts as a gateway, opening micro-channels through which
sodium ions travel. The sodium ion movement stimulates the release of glutamate. Glutamate in turn adjusts the polarity of the
neuron membranes, blocking or accessing further ion movement
between receptors. This causes the bleaching effect between color
determinants. The cone pigment itself is a protein called *iodopsin,*
which resonates with a molecule called *retinal* – a molecule derived
from vitamin A. When light hits the pigment, retinal's molecular
bonding structure changes from a *cis* configuration to a *trans* configuration. If we translate this oscillation to a static image, we might
imagine it being similar to the wing of an airplane being bent
downwards towards the ground. This *trans* configuration closes the
ion channel through a protein messenger called *transducin.* When the
ion channel is blocked, the neural signaling impulses are sent
through the optic nerve with a negative feedback of calcium ions.

Rather than initiating the flow of current, the stimulation of
light onto the cones *shuts off* the regular flow of ions through the
membrane. The concept of the *dark flow* – where a steady stream of
ions flow between these cells and the nerves is shut down when
stimulated by light – was reported in 1970 by Hagins *et al.*, from rod
pigments removed from the eyes of rats. This dark flow halting
process was evidenced through the measurement of tiny voltages
and currents among the photoreceptors.

What we are discussing then is a steady rhythmic current moving between the optic neurons, only to be intruded upon with the
reception of light through retinal cells. When our eyes are closed or
we are walking in pitch darkness, the rhythms flow. When light hits
the cones, a preponderance of retinal pigments stimulate particular
waveforms. These intercept and shut down the ion channels. This
interception process of shutting off the ion channels is called *hyper-
polarization* (Nakatani and Yau 1988).

The photocurrents running between the retinal cells and the
brain have specific waveform frequencies. These are classified as
alpha waves, beta waves and so on (Breton and Montzka 1992).
This classification of waveforms is defined by the orientation of
the brain wave oscillation frequencies that pulse through the brain.
The interaction between these *visual reception waves* and the other

oscillating rhythms circulating around the brain's neurons integrates visual perception into the mind's web, enabling a reflective picture to be observed by the self.

Note that this image reflected onto the mindscreen is not the actual image. It is a composite of colors, expectations, and a process of filling in the blanks. This filling in process creates a unique visual experience for each person. Though we may compare and confirm that we are all seeing some of the basic transmissions, each of us brings together a slightly different impression. This differential allows each of us an interpretive element, infusing our individual goals and objectives into the scene. This is why many people can watch the same show and notice different things. Perception is not an automated process. It is an act of consciousness.

As further evidence of this, in 1999 the *Proceedings of the National Academy of Sciences* published a study out of Stanford University firmly establishing that speaking the names of colors invokes the same brainwave response in subjects as the seeing of those colors (Suppes *et al.* 1999). Upon hearing a word describing a color, the brain triggers a translation into a mental image. The perception by the observer or conscious self makes no distinction between the sources of the input.

Color Therapy

Research has continued to connect the visual perception of color and brainwave response to our moods and behavior. Brain imaging has indicated that color stimulates corresponding brainwave patterns, which have been linked with particular moods and behaviors. The ancient science of Ayurveda correlates colors with particular energy states and subsequently, different *chakras* and energy centers around the body. The mechanism for this subtle electromagnetic bridge is explained using wave resonance and interference. If we were to hit a piano key in a room full of pianos, the other pianos would begin to vibrate in the same chord. With color resonance, we can associate particular waveforms with other oscillations occurring within the body. After all, colors are part of the electromagnetic wave spectrum. As these waveforms connect with our body in some respect, they stimulate internal waveform responses – just as touching a hot burner stimulates an immediate nervous response to pull our hand away.

Here is a review of the major colors. Some of this information comes from research, and some from traditional sources.

Red's longer wavelengths tend to stimulate higher frequency beta waves in the brain, vibrating at more than thirteen cycles per second with wavelengths of 630-700 nanometers. Its longer wavelength is responsible for the redness of the sunset. The longer wavelengths scatter less than the blues and violet waves as they interact with the atmosphere particles. Red tends to stimulate the body's autonomic systems, increasing heart rate and blood pressure.

The shorter (brighter) wavelengths of red will suppress melatonin release (Hanifin *et al.* 2006). However, longer-wave (darker) red colors have been shown to aid sleep and even induce melatonin. This latter effect has prompted some small studies showing that sleeping quality may be increased with periodic low-intensity red light. Other studies have shown that red light therapy restores glutathione balance, stimulates the immune system and improves wound healing (Yeager *et al.* 2006).

Traditional therapy indicates that red stimulates physical stamina, circulation, hostility, violence, competition, and jealousy. It also is considered stimulating to sexual activity. For this reason, a bright red dress or red roses often stimulates passion between the opposite sexes. It also seems to make sense that we find passionate people or very active people wearing reds and driving red cars. Red cars also tend to receive more speeding tickets. Whether this is because red car drivers drive faster or red cars are more noticeable is debatable. Red has been attributed to the planet mars, known for its connection to war, passion, and the struggle for survival. While red can be stimulating and aggressive, it is known to help relieve chronic pain. It also can stimulate the circulatory system and the liver. Because it stimulates greater stamina, red is considered helpful for completing projects requiring great amounts of physical energy and focus.

Orange tends to stimulate high alpha brainwaves, which oscillate between ten cycles per second and thirteen cycles per second at wavelengths of 590 to 630 nanometers. Orange has many of the stimulatory effects of red, but without some of the intensity and passion. Orange is therefore warming and anti-congestive. It is known to stimulate the lungs. It promotes enthusiasm, creativity, and inquisitiveness. Orange is often accompanied by sincerity, thoughtfulness, and health. Orange resonates with the sacral area – the back and lower spine – and the lower abdominal area according to *Ayurveda*. Orange stimulates reproductive activity – as opposed to the sexual passion of red. It also stimulates appetite and the movement of the colon. Orange resonates with aspects of family and parenting. Orange is also associated with wisdom and enlightenment. Activities that resonate the most with orange include family relationships, friendships and group organizations.

Yellow stimulates lower alpha brainwaves, eight or nine cycles per second with wavelengths of 560 to 590 nanometers. Yellow is known to stimulate the digestive tract. It is associated with the capacities of the stomach and upper intestines. Yellow also stimulates the adrenal glands. Thus, yellow is considered a trigger for stress. Activities associated with yellow include hyperactivity, memorization, study, and focus. For these reasons, yellow is also considered draining. Because yellow stimulates the adrenals, it can also stress the body and mind through the corticosteroids that it produces. Yellow resonates with spontaneity, compassion, memory, learning, and appetite. Yellow also reflects light with a greater intensity, so it can be exhausting on the eyes and mind after some time. This intensity can also stimulate digestion and nutrient assimilation, however. Yellow can be cheerful, but too much of it can be fatiguing. In behavioral research, yellow rooms seem to cause more anxiety. Babies cry more and couples argue more in yellow rooms.

Green stimulates brainwaves in the higher theta region, about six to seven cycles per second with a wavelength of 490 to 560 nanometers. Green is calming and balancing. It stimulates growth, love and a sense of security. Green resonates with the pituitary gland and is thus good for strengthening the endocrine system and regulating hormones. It tends to reduce blood pressure and congestion. It is also connected to devotion and giving. Green is soothing, yet it stimulates the immune system. It stimulates the activities of the thymus gland. Thus, green is considered a healing color. This is consistent with the fact that most green foods are immunostimulating and detoxifying. The green frequencies of light tend to suppress the body's endogenous melatonin levels. In a study from the U.K.'s

Loughborough University (Horne *et al.* 1991), six sleep-deprived human subjects were given 10 minutes of green light per hour in the evening, resulting in more alertness, less sleepiness and lower melatonin levels. This, combined with green's calming nature tends to help increase focus and alertness. The greens of nature's forests and gardens are testimony of green's ability to bring about calm focus. This effect is why green packaging is a favorite among consumers. Green radiation is also associated with problem-solving, negotiation, resolution, gardening and cooking.

Green may also help relieve depression. In a study at the University of California-San Diego (Loving *et al.* 2005), 33 elderly human subjects with depression were given bright green light for one hour per day or dim red light as a placebo. Mood improved for 23% of all the green-light subjects. Another study showed that green light slowed high frequency heart rate variability (Schäfer and Kratky 2006).

Blue stimulates lower theta waves in the five to six hertz area at wavelengths of 450 to 490 nanometers. Blue is cooling and calming. It slows metabolism. The rhythm of blue is gentle and holistic. Blue is associated with creativity and communication on both a spiritual and physical level. Like green, blue wavelengths help lower melatonin as the body increases adrenal hormones in the early part of the day. Blue activity is associated with relaxation, playing music and cleanliness. For this reason blue is associated with purification. Blue is also considered a color of stability and conservatism. Corporate executives and government administrators often choose blue for this reason. Blue is also a very good color to use around children, as it is calming and increases focus. In a study of 104 office workers, blue-enriched white light improved alertness, work performance and increased sleep quality (Viola *et al.* 2008). Schäfer and Kratky (2006) also showed that blue light significantly reduced heart rate variability. According to *Ayurveda*, blue resonates with breathing, speaking and the thyroid gland. The thyroid is the endocrine gland known to regulate body temperature and cellular metabolism.

Indigo stimulates low delta waves around one cycle per second and wavelengths of 400 to 450 nanometers. Therefore, indigo resonates with deep thinking, clarity, intuition and intelligence. It is a color linked with decision-making and meditative thinking. The sinuses, vision, and the immune system are therefore stimulated by indigo. Activities traditionally associated with indigo include highly intellectual activity, humanitarian behavior, medical research, and philosophical contemplation. It is a color is often associated with exploring the reason for existence.

Violet stimulates higher delta waves from two to four hertz. These waves vibrate at a faster frequency than indigo, primarily because they are more stimulating. Violet has been traditionally associated with raising consciousness and stimulating spiritual quests. Violet is also associated with nerve conduction, brain circulation, spinal fluid movement, and synovial fluid condition. Violet activities are associated with deep meditation and inspiration, prayer, and spiritual insight.

Purple, a color blending the effects of indigo and violet, is associated with luxury, royalty and nobility. It is considered a favorite of the wealthy and political-powerful, as it expresses feelings of superiority and dignity.

Research indicates blended colors have yet their own unique effects.

Pink has been associated with sedative and muscle-relaxing effects. Behavioral therapists like Alexander Schauss, Ph.D. have reported that pink colors create a tranquilizing effect, preventing or slowing anger and anxiety. Surprisingly, Dr. Schauss also reported this same effect among colorblind patients.

Light blue seems to bring about better mental performance. This relates to not only the calming effects of blue. The softness of the color stimulates intellectual cognition.

Black is a shade and not a color. Still, black appears to influence seriousness and even depression. Former prisoners of the former Soviet Union have reported that the KGB utilized black cells to induce depression in their interrogations. Black is of course the color most associated with death, as it is worn at funerals. Other black clothing events (such as "black tie affairs") are associated with seriousness and the need to establish dominance and order. On a brighter note, black is also considered elegant and clear. Black clothing or black automobiles may also reflect an intent to be conservative and uncomplicated. At the same time, black can also express boldness. Black is associated with both simply because black is an abrupt and muted waveform – it more clearly reflects the consciousness behind its use.

In general, colors with lower frequency and longer waveforms such as red, orange, and yellow tend to stimulate physical activity and resonate with physiological activities such as reproduction, survival, digestion, and thermal energy production. The higher frequency, shorter wavelength color waveforms of blue, violet, and indigo tend to stimulate brainwaves associated with thoughtfulness, problem solving, and intuition. Green is considered the crossover waveform, as it tends to bring balance among these activities.

When choosing colors to wear or otherwise surround our physical environment with, we might consider the goals we intend to achieve. The colors with the longest wavelengths such as red, yellow, and orange can be used when we need speed, energy, stamina, and immediate responses. When we need to be 'upbeat' about an activity or event, brighter colors will lift our mood and behavior. These brighter colors are also useful to fight depression and sluggishness. If we need to boost our enthusiasm, these brighter colors are significantly useful.

The cooler colors of violet, indigo, blue, and green will taper down and balance our energy levels. These colors will provide a relaxing meditative environment. We can let the stresses and the traumas slide right over us, as we surround ourselves with these colors. Certainly, it is quite easy to be surrounded by the greens and the blues of nature. All we have to do is take a walk in a natural environment with lots of green trees under a blue sky. This environment will stimulate greater intuition, problem solving, intelligence, and even possibly spiritual insight.

Food Colors

A significant amount of research has confirmed that the same pigments providing the color in foods also give those foods their nutritional and therapeutic value. For example, curcumin – a color pigment giving turmeric its yellow color – has been shown to enhance the immune system. Curcumin, for example, has been reported to stimulate the production of T cells, B cells, macrophages, neutrophils, and natural killer cells. Curcumin also downgrades inflammatory cytokines (Jagetia and Aggarwal 2007).

Color pigments are produced by plants from the sun and nutrients from the soil. Plants produce most of their color pigments as part of their immune response to viruses, bacteria and other challenges. Many pigments protect the plant from ultraviolet rays. They also provide great benefit to humans. Here are a few:

Red foods including tomatoes, watermelon, apples, strawberries, red raspberries and pink grapefruit contain nutrients such as lycopene and astaxanthin. These biochemical pigments have been associated with cancer prevention, healthy lungs, cardiovascular health, and prostrate health.

Orange foods including squash, carrots, oranges, papaya and mango contain alpha- and beta-carotenes as well as cryptoxanthins. These components convert and support nerve and sensory cells. They also stimulate enzyme processes, provide strong antioxidant activity and increase metabolism. For example, vitamin A is a frequent component in orange foods, which promotes metabolism, nerve transduction, and retinal cell health.

Yellow foods including yellow pears, bananas, corn and summer squash contain limonenes, luteins, carotenes and zeaxanthins – pigments that guard against cancer growth, assist in detoxification, provide antioxidants, inhibit atherosclerosis, and assist in cellular metabolism.

Green foods including wheat grass, mustard, onions, leafy greens, cruciferous vegetables and spirulina contain zeaxanthins, sulforaphanes, isoiocyanates, allyl sulfides, amino acids and vitamins such as K and C – which assist with liver function, DNA repair, cell metabolism, and cancer prevention among others.

Purple foods including grapes, cherries, cabbage, eggplant and various berries contain ellagic acid, anthocyanins, pomeratrol, pycnogenol and other polyphenols. These elements work conjunctively to inhibit bacteria growth, increase detoxification, prevent cancer growth and balance hormones.

Brown foods including whole grains, nuts and legumes contain good levels of amino acids, fatty acids, vitamin E and isoflavones such as lignans and phytoestrogens. They thus help modulate and regulate hormones, increase immune function, build proteins, nourish cell membranes and provide fiber. They also provide complex carbohydrates – precursors to serotonin and melatonin production.

Color Strategies

❋ **Color balance:** Throughout the day, we are provided with a rainbow of changing colors to balance and stimulate our energy levels. At daybreak, we can see the coming sun with a red-orange-amber hue, stimulating our physical energy. Through the later morning, the yellows of the sun's radiation help keep our focus and energy. The glowing mid-day sun lifts our mood and energy levels. It is important to journey outside for at least a few minutes during the middle of the day to receive these colors.

❋ **Living around plants:** A source of soothing and healing energy prevails amongst the greens of the plants and trees of nature. For this reason, we can be around plants, or surround our living environments with plants. If we cannot live in a rural area with lots of nature's plants and trees around us, we can bring plants and trees into our homes.

❋ **Look up:** The blueness of the sky can also provide a calming feeling, while increasing our imagination and creativity. Looking up at the sky periodically throughout the day can be extremely soothing to the mind and physical body. The blue sky also increases problem solving, so we can look up to the sky as we are considering a solution to an important problem.

❋ **Sunsets:** Near the end of the day – at around dusk – the sky can have an array of colors, reflecting the rays of the sun reflecting through more of the atmosphere. The post-sunset sky can turn purple, violet, and even indigo. These colors influence spiritual insight and thoughts of higher consciousness, as we ponder the meaning of our lives and our purpose. We may also experience increased reflective and meditative feelings – as darkness begins to fall and the sky becomes increasingly violet and indigo.

❋ **Take off the sunglasses:** Engaging this beautiful natural pallet of color within our physical lives can instantly vanish with one simple and innocent act: putting on a pair of sunglasses. Sunglasses can modulate a significant part of nature's visible spectrum. While this may be very convenient and even good for the eyes when we are driving with significant glare reflecting off other cars, there is a negative side effect as well: Sunglasses refract, polarize and diffuse light rays. They bring to the eyes unnatural and unreal colors. While some sunglasses may appear to brighten the colors around us, others remove light and colors and thus dampen color. Depressing color will depress our moods and cognition. Artificially brightening and changing the color pallet around us renders an ungrounded, almost eerie mood.

* **Worse are dark sunglasses:** Darker sunglasses can bring about even darker physiological and psychological effects. For one, the darkening of light depresses the pineal gland, which suppresses serotonin and dopamine secretion. These two important neurochemicals are critical for the balance of our moods and behavior. Depressing these secretions can result in feeling fatigued, depressed, and lethargic. Dark glasses can unnaturally raise melatonin levels. Increased melatonin stimulates sleepiness and lethargy. In the middle of the day – particularly while driving – this is not a good idea.

* **Even worse are automatic darkening eyeglasses.** Eyeglasses that automatically darken with increased light are convenient, and we can appreciate the advances in glass colorimetry. However, the problem with wearing automatically-darkening eyeglasses is that not only are we robbed of much of the light needed to stimulate important hormones and neurotransmitters and cheated of the benefit of natural colors: We are also entraining our bodies, nervous system and endocrine glands to a world of dampened color and reduced light. This entrainment might be compared to sending a person to live in a darkened cave. After awhile, they cannot deal with going outside into the light.

* **Pick your colors:** The colors of our rooms, our houses, our cars, and our clothing can all be chosen with the color effects mentioned. If we are going to a negotiation where

we want to communicate calmness, we might want to wear dark blue. Should we want to convey increased energy amongst our associates, we might wear some orange. Should we be seeking a balanced approach in our relationships we might consider wearing green.

* **Room color:** The walls of our rooms can affect cognition. Studies have shown that color photographs with natural scenery are remembered more than black and white photos, though unnaturally colored photos are remembered no better than black and white photos. Therefore, to enhance learning and memory, we can pick natural colors and images to surround ourselves with as much natural visual environment as possible. A natural visual environment might include, for example, a large picture window to a natural setting, an array of indoor plants, and natural fiber and wood furniture. A selection of nature's greens, blues, oranges and yellows can enhance our moods and promote relaxation. This in turn reduces the stress load upon the body.

* **Outdoor living:** By far the easiest way of accomplishing these results is to live in an outdoor or semi-outdoor environment for as much of the day and night as possible. This means opening our blinds and drapes as much as possible to let the light of the sun and the colors produced by sunlight into our living space. If our house or building is not currently very accommodating in this respect, there are a couple of easy strategies to increase our exposure to nature's colors. If we are inclined for home improvement, we can enlarge our windows by replacing them with sliding doors. This allows increased light and color exposure, along with increased thermal exposure. If we cannot replace them, we can always sit closer to them. We can set our desks and beds next to those windows with more color exposure. A note of caution, however: We should not look at computers or TVs with the sun shining from behind them for any length of time. This can damage our retinas, possibly causing photosensitivity.

* **Landscaping:** Many of our yards are covered with mani-cured concrete and stones. Concrete looks nice and neat, but it is not good for our eyes. Pulling those stones and sur-rounding our houses with green plants is an easy way to get more green color into our eyes. Even those native plants we consider "weeds" offer therapeutic colors to us – along with various medicinal properties. Look for native plants that need little water. Brightly flowering plants are preferred. These plants will take care of our environments if we take care of them. Their roots will prevent erosion. Their leaves will mulch the soil, leaving healthy soil. When we are sick, we can make tea from their leaves (consult an herbalist or reference and be sure to carefully identify the plant first).

* **Choose the right house:** When we are looking for a new place to live, let the outside environment be one of the more important criteria. Look at the amount of trees around the house. Look at the views from each window. The more of nature's views are visible, and the less views of concrete or neighboring houses, the better. That house or apartment – surrounded more by nature – will offer us a less stressful and more creative environment to live within.

* **Color-bathing:** In general, surrounding ourselves with na-ture's colors, eating foods with nature's colors, and focusing our eyes upon nature's plants, waters and sky will leave us with greater creativity, enthusiasm, wisdom, enlightenment, and relaxation. We can consider nature's colors like a clean-sing bath. We should regularly and frequently bathe in nature's colors just as we might wash our hands or take a shower.

* **Open up:** The heck with privacy. Let's open all the win-dows, pull the blinds and open the curtains. Let's take off the sunglasses, remove the tinting, and see the colors that nature intended our eyes to see.

Chapter Seven

Sun Medicine

With all the warnings about the sun's harmful effects, we might consider the sun as more of a toxin than necessary for life. Today modern culture blocks the sun as if it were toxic enemy number one. Sunscreen, sunblock, sun cream, sunglasses, sun awnings, sunshades, sun umbrellas, sun tinting, sun canopies, and sun hats: Can the sun really be this dangerous?

And what were people doing before sun block came along? Did not most humans work primarily outside all day – in the fields growing and preparing food, washing clothes, bathing, and so on? Now as we sit indoors in front of our computers, for some reason the sun has suddenly become toxic.

Most humans have experienced the positive effects of sunlight. This is why humans tend to vacation in sunny areas. A vacation to a tropical or sunny destination typically results in increased feelings of well-being and relaxation. Many also experience a decrease in allergies, headaches, joint pain and backaches. While there is certainly the element of relaxation and lowered stress during vacation, it is unmistakable: Sunlight contributes to the health of the body.

The sun's resonating energies deliver heat and raise core body temperature. Higher core body temperatures increase cell function. This increases metabolism, facilitating detoxification. Boosted core temperatures regulate the levels of cortisol and melatonin, which balance our sleep and energy levels.

Sun also regulates our natural biorhythm cycles. The sun's waveforms stimulate the body's pineal gland, synchronizing the body's clockworks triggered through the suprachiasmatic nuclei cells. These SCN cells mark the passage of time for the body, regulating the body's metabolic functions. A day without sunlight will leave the body's cells confused. This is illustrated by the common experience of disorientation after sleeping in late on a Saturday morning. On an extended basis, a day without a good portion of natural sunlight – even if just seen through a window screen – will leave the body's natural rhythms in a state of disarray.

The reception and absence of sunlight stimulates the pineal gland's production of melatonin, which regulates sleep and body core temperature. Melatonin also plays a major role in the immune system. The pineal gland stimulates the hypothalamus to release neurotransmitters, which stimulate the anterior pituitary gland. The pituitary then releases master hormones that drive our body's endocrine system.

Much of the nutritional energy utilized by life on this planet comes through the thin leaves of plants: via a mechanism called photosynthesis. Through microscopic pores in the leaf called *stomata*, the plant absorbs carbon dioxide. From the roots below, water is absorbed and brought through tiny veins to the leaf. Tiny *chloroblasts* of multiple chlorophyll molecules drink specific rays of the sun, utilizing those waveforms to split water into hydrogen and oxygen atoms. The resulting hydrogen atoms combine with carbon dioxide to form carbohydrates (CH_2O, to $C_6H_{12}O_6$), while oxygen atoms are released into the air. The carbohydrates form sugars, starches and cellulose within the plant, directly providing fuel to plant-eating species and indirectly providing fuel for those species that eat plant-eaters. None of this could be possible without the sun's radiation. It is the sun's violet-blue and lower red-orange wavelengths of the visible spectrum that plants primarily utilize. The green wavelengths are reflected back – giving the leaf its characteristic green color.

The molecular structure of the chlorophyll molecule is daisy-shaped – called a *porphyrin ring*. Its molecular shape almost precisely mirrors the radiant orb from which it converts energy. This ring-shaped chlorophyll structure (sometimes connected with the *phytol* chain) allows the radiation to freely migrate, enabling an electron transport process called *fluorescence resonance*. This energy transfer process converts specific wavelengths of radiation from the sun into excited orbitals within the molecule. The excited state is a constructive interference between the radiation waves from the sun and the bonding orbitals of the electrons (standing waves) within the chlorophyll molecule. This coherent interference creates an energy transfer chain very similar to the Krebs energy cycle occurring within our cells. Both are considered electron-transport cycles. As the electron-waves are transferred, NADP+ is reduced to NADPH, which enables the conversion of carbon dioxide to sugar – the fuel of choice for other organisms.

The process of photosynthesis is incredibly complex. We merely summarize it here. Within the process, there are many catalysts and nutrients gathered from the earth's soils, such as magnesium, which lies in the center of the porphyrin structure. Carotenoids assist in different ways. They buffer the process when too much radiation is involved, and they alleviate barriers to the process at lower levels of radiation. Phytochemicals such as phycobilins, ferredoxin, adenosine triphosphate and fucoxanthins facilitate the photosynthetic process. Other phytonutrients such as beta-carotene, alpha-carotene and alpha-tocopherol protect the plant from the effects of too much radiation. Vitamins like beta-carotene work in a similar way inside our bodies – protecting our cells from radiation damage.

About three-quarters of this planet's photosynthesis takes place within the oceans, thus involving the *Cyanobacteria* and *Rhodophyta* families of the plant kingdom. Quite simply, the complexity of photosynthesis and its ability to provide the fuel needed for life is a miraculous array of waveform precision and design. The sun is a needed element for the health of every living creature – large and small.

The sun is also our medicine.

A Prescriptive Sun

The sun has been used as a medicine for many centuries. It has been a central healing agent in the world's oldest medicine, *Ayurveda*. The sun was described as a prescriptive agent in the ancient Egyptian medical text, the *Ebers Papyrus*. It has been a central component for North and South American and Polynesian native tribes. It has been a key element used in Traditional Chinese Medicine. The Greeks and Romans both used sun cures for many infectious diseases such as **tuberculosis.** Hippocrates was a big proponent for the use of sunbathing treatments for a number of illnesses. In later centuries, large healing centers have been erected for the purpose of healing with the sun. The Nords, Scots, Irish, Aborigines, Iranians, Assyrians, Japanese and Indonesians all treated disease with sunbathing.

For centuries, a devastating disease became prevalent in Europe, where bones would twist and spindle. This seemed to arbitrarily attack children, sometimes fatally. This disease was termed *richettes* – a derivative of the word 'wretcheds.' It devastated Europe, especially in the winter. In the early 1800s, French physician Cauvain recommended sunlight for **rickets.** Controversial at first, this hypothesis was also published by the Polish physician Andrew Sniadecki in 1822. The theory was virtually ignored until the late nineteenth century. An English missionary physician named Theodor Palm, while traveling in the east, realized the connection between rickets and sunlight and advocated sunlight for the prevention of rickets. This treatment was eventually adopted by Swiss physician August Rollier.

A century later, it was discovered that a combination of vitamin D from the sun, calcium, boron and phosphate work together to form bone tissue cells, or osteocytes. Without enough sunlight, not enough vitamin D will be produced, leaving the bones unformed or maligned. Today this same disease has become relevant in the form of **osteoporosis** and **osteomyalgia.**

As modern-day adults age, they are spending less and less time outside. With less vitamin D production, bones become weaker. **Hip fractures** and other bone breakages become common. This is well documented. Over ten million people in the U.S. now have osteoporosis. More have **osteopenia,** which puts them at risk of osteoporosis and bone fractures. Research has shown that about 50% of women and 25% of men over the age of fifty will suffer an osteoporosis-related fracture.

Swiss physician Dr. Arnold Rikli was considered one of the earliest modern proponents of sunbathing as medicine during the nineteenth century. Dr. Rikli propounded what he called *atmospheric healing,* which included open-air sunbathing, nighttime open-air huts, water treatments, barefoot walking and constant fresh air. Dr. Rikli established a famous health clinic in Bled, Slovenia. People traveled from around Europe to his center, and many found success with his treatments for many years. Rikli himself, a vegetarian, naturalist, and early naturopath, lived to the ripe age of 97. His open-air sun treatments are still referred to as the *Rikli Cure.*

In the 1860s, Dr. Hermann Brehmer was successful in treating tuberculosis and other infections with open-air sunlight in a German sanatorium. Dr. Brehmer himself was diagnosed with tuberculosis, and was cured using his treatments. His healing center is said to have contained over 300 beds, and his tuberculosis sun cure was considered the most successful tuberculosis treatment to date.

Dr. Dio Lewis was also a leading sunlight expert. He documented treating **rheumatic diseases, dyspepsia, neuralgia,** and other diseases with great success using sunbathing in a book entitled *Weak Lungs and How to Make Them Strong* (1863).

Dr. James Jackson, in his book, *How to Treat the Sick Without Drugs* (1868) documented treating up to 125 patients with sunbathing. He commented that even those who had failed various other conventional treatments were significantly *"strengthened and innervated."* He commented that patients who had trouble sleeping were able to not only fall asleep, but also able to nap outside. His conclusion was that sunlight was one of the most therapeutic agents known to him and his peers of the day.

Dr. Niels Finsen was awarded the 1903 Nobel Prize in medicine for revealing that sunshine was extremely therapeutic for a number of **infectious diseases,** including **lupus vulgaris, small pox,** and **Pick's disease.** Dr. Finsen's famous sunbaths and separated light colors became known as *Finsen Light Therapy.*

In the early 1900s, two Swiss physicians Dr. Oskar Bernhard and Dr. Rollier found that the sun in thin atmospheres such as the Swiss Alps provided an effective therapeutic protocol for **surgical tuberculosis** and **lung tuberculosis.** Sunlight has since been shown effective as a part of treatment for various other conditions.

Dr. Benedict Lust, considered the father of American naturopathic medicine, prescribed sunbathing treatment for various **degenerative diseases.** Dr. Lust's nude sunbathing treatments were considered radical by federal and state authorities.

Dr. Jethro Kloss and Dr. John Harvey Kellogg were also physicians held in high esteem and national recognition for their various naturopathic therapies. Both had popular treatment centers, also called sanitariums, in which they utilized sunbathing for a variety of disorders. Dr. Kellogg also used artificial sunlight treatments, which he called, together with sunlight treatment, *phototherapy.*

Dr. Herbert Shelton, in his book *The Hygienic System: Fasting and Sun Bathing* (1939) was also a physician with a significant amount of research and experience with sunbathing. Dr. Shelton prescribed sunshine for **heart disease, tuberculosis, asthma** and **nervous diseases.**

In a study by Dr. Fritz Hollwich (Hollwich and Dieckhues 1989), 110 cataract patients underwent metabolic testing before and after cataract opacity surgery. Prior to surgery, the opacity of their cataracts significantly reduced the amount of light to about 10% of normal. Testing prior to surgery showed **reduced metabolism, adrenal insufficiency** and **hormone imbalances.** After surgery – the removal of the lens opacities – metabolism and hormone levels returned to normal.

These results were confirmed with another study (Hollwich and Hartmann 1990) performed shortly thereafter on fifty cataract patients with the same results. This later study also looked at water balance, blood sugar and blood cell count – all of which improved following surgery and light. Dr. Hollwich describes the retino-hypothalamic pathway connecting the endocrine-visceral system.

Research has indicated that the visible light spectrum (400-700 nm) received from the sun through both the eyes and the skin increases the body's immune response. As light is received through the retina, its energy is delivered to the LGM and visual cortex through transduction while being delivered to the suprachiasmatic nucleus in the hypothalamus. This stimulates the release of hypo-thalamic-pituitary hormones. Light also stimulates the pineal gland directly, stimulating a cascade of hormones and neurotransmitters through the pituitary gland. Melatonin, norepinephrine, and acetyl-choline secretions (the latter two known for stress response) decrease, while cortisol, serotonin, GABA and dopamine secretions increase with increased sunlight. These latter three are noted for relaxation and calmness, while cortisol is related to **inflammation** reduction. All are related directly or indirectly to immune response.

Visible light also penetrates the epidermal and dermal skin layers, interacting directly with circulating lymphocytes. Sunlight thus increases immune cell responsiveness, which allows the body to defend itself against **practically every pathogen and toxin** currently known (Roberts 2000).

Ultraviolet-A in particular has been shown to directly assist the immune system by aiding the repair of **DNA damage**. This effect was illustrated in a series of studies on tiny unicellular paramecia led by Dr. Joan Smith-Sonneborn, a University of Wyoming professor. While bursts of unscreened ultraviolet-C caused DNA damage, ultraviolet-A exposure reversed the damage. Going beyond the reversal of genetic damage, additional exposure to ultraviolet-A radiation extended the paramecia's life span as much as fifty percent (Smith-Sonneborn 1979; Rodermel and Smith-Sonneborn 1977).

The sun is also an effective antiseptic. Various studies have shown the sun to be antimicrobial in many respects. Many **pathogenic bacteria** and **fungi** are intolerant to the rays of the sun. Some are overheated by the sun's thermal rays. Many others are destroyed by the sun's infrared radiation (Piluso and Moffat-Smith 2006). These include certain molds and bacteria, which can significantly multiply in a dark, wet environment.

In a review of various cardiovascular system studies from the Department of Medicine of the University of Alabama (Rostand 1997), a correlation between ultraviolet radiation and **blood pressure** was reported. In multiple studies, blood pressure rises among populations with increased distance from the equator. In other words, increased sun exposure decreases blood pressure. This report also correlated the increased hypertension rates among northern populations of darker skin and higher melanin content. Because melanin levels block ultraviolet rays, darker skin types require more sun exposure to reach the same level of benefit from the sun.

Hypertension is not the only heart disease-related issue that has been connected to decreased sun exposure. The Cardiovascular Thrombosis Research Center from the University of Massachusetts Medical Center (Spencer *et al.* 1998) studied 259,891 cases of **myocardial infarction**. After adjusting for controls and standardized seasons, it was found there were 53% more heart attacks reported in the winter than in the summer. Fatalities also followed a similar seasonal pattern. Another study done at Australia's Monash University in 2008 (Loughnan *et al.*) of 33,165 myocardial infarction over 2,186 consecutive days showed a definite peak in the colder months, with a peak among men of 33.7% increased heart attacks during winter months.

Multiple studies have shown vitamin D deficiency present in a majority of **congestive heart failure** cases (Zittermann 2006). It is not hard to link other **heart** and **cardiovascular diseases** to a lack of sunshine from the research.

In fact, a significant amount of research over the past few decades has linked a lack of sunshine to many other diseases. In addition to the ones mentioned above, there are many others, including **multiple sclerosis, rheumatoid arthritis, Crohn's disease, irritable bowel syndrome, acne, psoriasis, jaundice, depression, eczema, high blood pressure, heart disease, diabetes, hypothyroidism, angina, prostate cancer, lung cancer, colon cancer, ovary cancer, kidney disease, hyperparathyroidism, uterine cancer, stomach cancer, kidney cancer, lymphoma, pancreatic cancer, ovarian cancer, tooth loss, bone loss, obesity, joint inflammation, insomnia, Parkinson's disease, fibromyalgia** and a variety of **immune-** and **autoimmune-related diseases** (Cuppari and Garcia-Lopes 2009, Egan *et al.* 2005, Giovannucci 2005, Holick 2004, McCarty 2003).

Vitamin D and Melanin

It is now well known from the research that the sun's ultraviolet-B rays stimulate our bodies to synthesize vitamin D_3. Vitamin D is more of a hormone than a vitamin. It is a critical biochemical for the body, as we will discuss. The hormone-vitamin D_3 molecule is produced when ultraviolet-B in wavelengths of 270-290 nanometers enters our epidermis. Here a derivative of cholesterol called *7-dehydrocholesterol* undergoes a *conrotatory electrocyclic reaction* to produce a pre-vitamin D. The pre-vitamin D molecule undergoes hydroxylation in the liver and kidneys to convert to the final D_3 structure – 1,25 dihydroxyvitamin D (some refer to this as 25-OHD). The conrotary reaction illustrates a synchronous circular waveform reaction, as atoms and their bonds rotate around the ring.

Within a 7-dehydrocholesterol-saturated biomolecular environment of the epidermis, specialized cells called *melanocytes* produce a protective biochemical called *melanin*. Skin melanocytes are primarily located at the lower strata of the epidermis. Other melanocytes located around the body produce specialized forms of melanin. Melanocytes within the uvea, which contains the iris, produce the melanin that gives the color to our irises. Melanocytes around our hair follicles give color to our hair. Melanocytes within the leptomeninges residing within our brain and spinal cord produce a type of melanin thought to support cerebrospinal fluid circulation.

Melanin is produced through an enzymatic process involving the amino acid tyrosine. This process takes place within small sacs inside the melanocytes called *melanosomes*. Two types of melanin may be produced, depending upon the location and production stimulated: *Eumelanin* has a black or brown tint. *Pheomelanin* has a reddish or yellowish tint. Depending upon our genetic information, our body may produce more of one type of melanin than another, producing the color features of our skin, hair and eyes.

Once produced in skin melanocytes, melanin is transferred to the keratinocytes, which lie on the external skin barrier. Melanin is the biochemical pigment that makes the skin turn brown. Melanin also provides a natural sunscreen for the skin: The greater the melanin level, the fewer ultraviolet-B rays reach the 7-dehydrocholesterol molecules, and the less vitamin D_3 is produced. Vitamin D is used in thousands of metabolic processes around the body. What is not used is stored within fat cells for later use.

Natural vitamin D from the sun is extremely important to all of the body's tissues – and an essential part of the immune system. Vitamin D is most known to regulate calcium levels and absorption. Without proper vitamin D_3 production, calcium will not be absorbed into our bones and teeth. For this reason, osteoporosis and other joint problems are becoming more commonplace in modern society. Vitamin D is also critically important for healthy immune function, nervous function, cardiovascular health, mood regulation, pain regulation, insulin/blood sugar balance, as well as numerous endocrine and digestive functions. Vitamin D is a necessary component for good health, and its most natural form (D_3) comes from natural sun exposure (Lehmann 2005).

Because vitamin D_2 will also convert to 1,25 dihydroxyvitamin D, it was assumed until recently that D_2 and D_3 were functionally identical within the body. This assumption has since been proven incorrect. In a study done at the Creighton University and the Medical University of South Carolina (Armas *et al.* 2004), twenty healthy males were measured following supplementation of either

D_2 or D_3. While both converted to 1,25 dihydroxyvitamin D, D_2 converted at far lower levels and even those levels fell off more quickly. The study's authors concluded that D_2 has only about one-third the potency of D_3.

In a Boston University study published in 2008, forty-five nursing home patients took a multivitamin containing 400 IU of vitamin D_2. During the study period, their 25-OHD levels registered deficient from a range of 49% to 78% in measurements over an eight-month period.

A 1998 study (Thomas *et al.*) of 290 medical ward patients at the Massachusetts General Hospital in Boston showed that 57% were vitamin D deficient (164) and 65 of those (22%) were severely deficient. Surprisingly, 46% were deficient despite taking the recommended dosage of vitamin D. The elderly and those in **pain** are most often vitamin D deficient. One study (Al Faraj and Al Mutairi 2003) found that 83% of 360 **low-back pain** patients had vitamin D deficiency. Another (Plotnikoff and Quigley 2003) showed that 93% of 150 nonspecific pain patients had vitamin D deficiency. In this latter study, nearly all of those patients declared pain relief after three months of vitamin D supplementation, and in the former study, – of the 360 low-back pain patients – 95% showed clinical improvement after treatment with supplemental vitamin D_3.

Chronic kidney disease is also more prevalent among those deficient in vitamin D (Khan 2007). Vitamin D deficiency was linked to tuberculosis by Sita-Lumsden *et al.* in 2007. Vitamin D has also been shown to protect against **macular degeneration** by Parekh in 2007. **Cognition, mania, depression** and other **mood related disorders** are also linked with vitamin D deficiency (Berk *et al.* 2007). Vitamin D deficiency was linked to a higher incidence of **osteoporosis** by Barone (*et al.* 2007). **Fetal diabetes, pre-eclampsia** and **fetal neurological disorders** were connected to vitamin D deficiency by Perez-Lopez in 2007. Serum vitamin D was also connected with higher **insulin sensitivity** by Kamycheva *et al.* in 2007.

Vitamin D, when taken together with calcium, was linked to better glucose metabolism by Pittas *et al.* in 2007. In a Creighton University study (Lappe *et al.* 2007) of 1179 postmenopausal women, cancer rates among those supplementing with calcium and vitamin D_3 had an almost 60% lower **cancer** rate than the control subjects. A number of cancers are apparently prevented or ameliorated by vitamin D.

These are but a few of the hundreds of clinical studies confirming at last count, that over **70 disorders** are linked with vitamin D deficiency!

Is Supplemented Vitamin D Really Therapeutic?

Research linking vitamin D deficiency to disease has all but brought the medical industry and health media to a standing ovation. Vitamin D has been heralded as the world's most important vitamin – even though it is more of a hormone than a vitamin.

And truly, vitamin D deficiency has now been linked to dozens of medical conditions in the research, including insomnia, hypertension, arthritis, asthma, autism, low-back pain, Parkinson's disease, multiple sclerosis, heart and cardiovascular disease, chronic fatigue, tuberculosis, Crohn's disease, neuropathy, osteoporosis, diabetes, heart disease, cancer, liver disease, mental disorders, different cancers and other conditions.

The assumption has been that since deficiency is linked to these diseases, removing the deficiency with supplementation should vastly reduce these conditions. Right? Not so fast.

A large review of research (Autier *et al.* 2014) published in the British Medical Association journal Lancet – analyzed 290 clinical studies that examined vitamin D deficiency, and 172 clinical studies for disease outcomes. The research comes from the International Prevention Research Institute in Lyons, France.

Indeed, the study found significant *("moderate to strong")* associations between vitamin D *deficiency* and:

"cardiovascular diseases, serum lipid concentrations, inflammation, glucose metabolism disorders, weight gain, infectious diseases, multiple sclerosis, mood disorders, declining cognitive function, impaired physical functioning, and all-cause mortality."

However, the research did not find associations between higher vitamin D levels in the blood and cancer outside of colorectal cancer.

Okay, so maybe vitamin D deficiency isn't associated with all the conditions mentioned above, but enough to be important. Heart disease? Multiple sclerosis? Mortality? Cognitive function? Yes, vitamin D is critical.

But the blockbuster of the study was that even though deficiency was linked to all those conditions, supplementation did not have a therapeutic effect on any disease.

The researchers analyzed 34 "intervention" studies – studies that tested vitamin D supplementation using some form of randomization – amongst those with many of the conditions listed above.

The researchers stated that:

"Results from intervention studies did not show an effect of vitamin D supplementation on disease occurrence, including colorectal cancer."

The supplementation studies utilized vitamin D at levels greater than 50 micrograms per day – equivalent to 2,000 IU of vitamin D. But the researchers added that those studies using less than 2,000 IU didn't fare any better:

"In 34 intervention studies including 2805 individuals with mean 25(OH)D concentration lower than 50 nmol/L at baseline supplementation with 50 μg per day or more did not show better results."

Another blow to the notion that vitamin D supplementation is the magic cure for so many conditions is research negating the assumption that vitamin D supplementation will decrease bone density.

University of Auckland researchers (Reid *et al.* 2014) – funded by Health Research Council of New Zealand – found that vitamin D supplementation has little benefit to bone density of elderly persons. The study is published in January 2014's issue of the British Medical Journal *Lancet*.

This effect of vitamin D – that it increases bone density due to its synergistic relationship with calcium – has been one of the bedrocks upon which the need for vitamin D supplementation has been laid.

Using the Cochrane Database and Cochran's Q meta-analysis calculations, the New Zealand researchers reviewed 23 clinical studies that measured the effects of vitamin D supplementation on bone density. Out of these, only one study showed benefit for more than one site. And among all the studies, the meta-analysis showed no effects at any site with the exception of a small effect at the femoral neck region.

This result dealt a significant blow to the general recommendation that elderly persons should supplement with vitamin D to help prevent osteoporosis.

The researchers concluded:

"Continuing widespread use of vitamin D for osteoporosis prevention in community-dwelling adults without specific risk factors for vitamin D deficiency seems to be inappropriate."

Note they suggest *"without risk factors for vitamin D deficiency"* here. They are suggesting that supplementation for vitamin D deficiency is still recommended.

But is this correct? Is vitamin D a chicken-and-egg problem?

In trying to explain these odd results, the French researchers concluded that low levels of vitamin D were the result of ill health and inflammatory processes. Their conclusion is that aging and ill health causes vitamin D deficiency instead of the other way around:

"The discrepancy between observational and intervention studies suggests that low 25(OH)D is a marker of ill health. Inflammatory processes involved in disease occurrence and clinical course would reduce 25(OH)D, which would explain why low vitamin D status is reported in a wide range of disorders."

But the fact that some studies have shown that vitamin D supplementation can help reduce mortality and a few other conditions caused the researchers to back away from the hard line:

"In elderly people, restoration of vitamin D deficits due to ageing and lifestyle changes induced by ill health could explain why low-dose supplementation leads to slight gains in survival."

And it wasn't as if the supplementation in these studies didn't increase blood levels of 25-hydroxyvitamin D (25(OH)D) – the generic calciferol measurement that doesn't differentiate between the types of vitamin D (as we'll discuss below).

Certainly their conclusion has its merits. However, before we throw the baby out with the bath water on supplemented vitamin D, there are a few other issues to consider.

Is it possible that the forms of vitamin D being supplemented in most of these trials is the issue?

A study by researchers from France's International Prevention Research Institute (Autier *et al.* 2012) conducted a meta-analysis of studies that compared blood-levels of 25-hydroxyvitamin D that resulted from the supplementation of either vitamin D2 or vitamin D3, among those over the age of 50. They found 76 clinical studies between 1984 and 2011 that measured these.

The researchers found that vitamin D2 (ergocalciferol) and supplementation of vitamin D3 (cholecalciferol) did increase blood-levels of 25-hydroxyvitamin D (25(OH)D), but the D2 supplementation increased 25(OH)D levels significantly less.

Another study, this from the UK's University of Surrey (Heaney *et al.* 2011) also found that D2 increased blood levels of 25(OH)D significantly less than did D3. They concluded:

"This meta-analysis indicates that vitamin D3 is more efficacious at raising serum 25(OH)D concentrations than is vitamin D2, and thus vitamin D3) could potentially become the preferred choice for supplementation."

But blood levels of 25(OH)D aren't the only issues to consider. And certainly it isn't the bigger issue, as most of the studies in the *Lancet's* French review above did show significantly higher blood levels of 25(OH)D among those receiving the vitamin D supplementation – regardless of whether the supplement was D2 or D3.

But then the physiology runs deeper, as it relates to vitamin D receptors and the fact that the steps that eventually convert calciferol to calcitriol favor the physiologically-produced calciferol – sulfated-25(OH)D3 – through a process called hydroxylation.

"Data suggested that these proposed differences between the 2 calciferols are due to their differing affinities for the vitamin D receptor (VDR), which appears to be linked to an additional step of 24-hydroxylation that inactivates calcitriol. In addition, it is thought that vitamin D3 is potentially the preferred substrate for hepatic 25-hydroxylase, which in combination with the possible difference in the 24-hydroxylation rate, only reinforces the importance of determining whether these metabolic anomalies impact on health."

The last statement is critical, as both supplemented versions of vitamin D – vitamin D2 (ergocalciferol) and supplemented vitamin D3 (cholecalciferol) – are both analogs of the real vitamin D3 used by the body – 25-Hydroxyvitamin D3-3-beta-sulphate, also referred to as 25(OH)D3-sulfate. This is converted from 7-dehydrocholesterol and the sun's UVB rays.

The liver converts cholecalciferol from the blood to calcifediol. Calcifediol is then converted to calcitriol in the kidneys. Calcitriol is the biologically active form of vitamin D. If this is inactivated during D2 conversion (from the extra hydroxylation step) as the researchers note, then this is like taking two steps forward and three steps backward.

When doctors and researchers measure vitamin D levels in the blood, they don't measure calcitriol levels. They measure the assumed precursors – 25(OH)D in all its various forms, which include 25(OH)D2 (ergocalciferol) and 25(OH)D3 (cholecalciferol).

Furthermore, the ergocalciferol (D2) molecule is significantly different than cholecalciferol in that it has an additional methyl group on its 24th carbon. This is why it has to undergo that extra hydroxylation step in order to render calciferol.

But more importantly, as mentioned above, calcitriol becomes inactivated in this extra hydroxylation step. This means the process actually renders less available calcitriol – which the body utilizes, as it binds to cell receptors.

The critical issue is the binding of vitamin D in cells – Here is how the French researchers put it:

"First, vitamin D receptors have been found in various organs, and activation of these receptors by 1a,25 dihydroxyvitamin D3 (calcitriol), the physiologically active form of vitamin D, induces cell differentiation and inhibits proliferation, invasiveness, angiogenesis, and metastatic potential."

But as noted, the the conversion from ergocalciferol removes calcitriol. This is why D2 has also been shown to render far less sustainable vitamin D activity:

"This differentiation between ergocalciferol and cholecalciferol is due to the fact that once 1,24,25(OH)3D2 has been formed, ergocalciferol has been deactivated and, therefore, is irretrievable. In contrast, cholecalciferol [now 1,24,25(OH)3D3] retains its capacity to bind to the VDR [vitamin D receptors] and still requires an additional side-chain oxidation to become deactivated. Thus, this additional step gives a vast advantage and potential for cholecalciferol to remain biologically active and, thus, maintain vitamin D status, which only strengthen the hypothesis that cholecalciferol is the preferred substrate compared with ergocalciferol."

The statement *"to remain biologically active"* is precisely at issue when it comes to the research showing the poor therapeutic results of vitamin D supplementation (typically D2).

And even after vitamin D2 is converted to 25(OH)D in the blood, it is not sustainable. It does not readily convert to calcitriol. This was confirmed in a study by researchers from Nebraska's Creighton University. The researchers gave 50,000 IU per week of either D2 or D3 to 33 healthy adults for four months. They tested the subjects' 25-hydroxyvitamin D [25(OH)D] as well as their change in calciferol levels within subcutaneous fat cells – a measure of the body's retention and utilization of the vitamin D.

Yes, D3 was better retained in the blood, but D2 was also retained as 25(OH)D2. The researchers found that the 25(OH)D blood levels of those taking the D3 were nearly double those who took the D2 – 45 ng/ml versus 24 ng/ml.

Even more revealing was that calciferol levels within subcutaneous fat cells increased by 104 micrograms per kilogram among those taking D3, yet only increased by a measly .033 micrograms per kilogram (33 nanograms per kilogram) among those taking the D2. This means that the amount of vitamin D that reached the cells with D2 supplementation was 0.0031% – or 0.000031 – less than D3.

The researchers calculated that D3 supplementation is 87% *"more potent in raising and maintaining serum 25(OH)D concentrations and produces 2- to 3-fold greater storage of vitamin D than does equimolar D2."*

This was emphasized in a similar study (Tripkovic *et al.* 2012):

"When the evidence from the studies that focused on vitamin D metabolism at the cellular level is compared with the evidence from clinical trials, it is clear that, overall, there was consistency in the results that shows cholecalciferol appears to have advantageous biological qualities that allows it to sustain its systemic influence for far longer and at far greater concentrations than does ergocalciferol."

But as far as sustained bioactivity – its final storage within fat cells, the researchers concluded that neither supplementation program resulted in significant accumulation among fat cells:

"For neither was there evidence of sequestration in fat, as had been postulated for doses in this range."

This last point brings up the question of whether D2 supplementation – and possibly even supplemented D3 – is even therapeutic.

And while the research showing little benefit of vitamin D supplementation utilized studies that utilized vitamin D2 – many also utilized supplemented vitamin D3.

Furthermore, the characterization that vitamin D deficiency is linked to osteoporosis, cardiovascular disease, cancers and many other conditions has been determined by linking vitamin D deficiency with these conditions. This means that the question that has yet to be proven is whether vitamin D supplementation with synthetic forms – especially D2 and possibly even D3 – will reverse the type of vitamin D deficiencies linked among these conditions.

The shocker is that vitamin D2 supplementation will actually reduce the more biologically active form of vitamin D3 in the blood. And by doing that, actually reduce vitamin D function in the body. If we combine this with the effect that even D3 supplementation doesn't sequester well within fat cells, we may have a problem with both supplemented D2 and D3.

In fact, vitamin D2 supplementation actually lowers levels of the physiologically active form of calciferol.

For six weeks, University of California researchers (Binkley and Eiebe 2013) gave 38 adult volunteers either mushrooms not treated with UV exposure (containing 34 IU of D per 100 grams), UV-treated mushrooms (containing from 352 to 684 IU per 100 grams), or a supplement containing 1000 IU of D2 along with untreated mushrooms. The researchers tested the blood levels of vitamin D2 and D3 (25(OH)D2 and 25(OH)D3) before and after the testing to determine whether the mushrooms and/or supplement was increasing the vitamin D status of the subjects.

Surprisingly, the researchers found that while their blood vitamin D2 (25(OH)D2) levels went up, their 25(OH)D3 levels went down about the same, leaving their net vitamin D levels about the same and not increased as one would assume from the supplementation.

The disturbing thing about this study comes when we blend the understanding from the other research that blood levels of 25(OH)D2 do not convert well to vitamin D-receptor synergistic calcitriol very well. This has led to the conclusion from the study above:

While ergocalciferol may push 25(OH)D2 levels up, 25(OH)D3 produced from cholecalciferol suffers, leaving little net gain.

The researchers confirmed this in their discussion:

"Thus, ergocalciferol intake from mushrooms is beneficial for participants at risk of deficiency but may not improve status cholecalciferol participants with considerable sun exposure and resulting cutaneous synthesis of cholecalciferol."

"Cutaneous synthesis of cholecalciferol" means the sulfated form of cholecalciferol.

Yes, we can now conclude that vitamin D2 is not so therapeutic and can even reduce our levels of the more therapeutic 25(OH)D3. But this issue of sulfated cholecalciferol is critical to the topic of whether vitamin D3 supplementation is therapeutic.

Synthetic forms of vitamin D3 are typically unsulfated forms of vitamin D, while the vitamin D produced by the sun is 25-Hydroxyvitamin D3 3 beta-sulphate. This is a water-soluble form of 25(OH)D3 – sometimes referred to as vitamin D3-sulfate.

Yes, the form of vitamin D3 from supplements is not conjugated with sulfate. Does this make a difference?

In fact, the research that discerned the difference between the sulfated and unsulfated forms tested 60 patients for serum levels of both (Axelson 1985). The research concluded:

"The study also shows that unconjugated 25-hydroxyvitamin D3 is not readily sulphated by man in vivo."

This certainly indicates that supplemented, unsulfated vitamin D3 form will likely not act the same within the body as does the body's own sulfated form of vitamin D3 produced from sunlight. And this likely explains the reason why the Creighton University researchers did not find significant fat cell sequestration from either D2 or D3 supplementation.

Yes, the sunlight-produced form of vitamin D3 – sulfated-D3 – is the most biologically active form of vitamin D. And because it is so biologically active, nature's form of vitamin D produced through UVB sunlight exposure is stored within the body in the form of fat cell sequestration. So we don't even need it every day. In fact, a good dose of UVB can allow the body to retain sufficient vitamin D for weeks, even a month or two with significant doses.

Remember the one bright star of the *Lancet* study above was that mortality was slightly reduced by vitamin D supplementation.

And this study result is mirrored by a 2007 review of 18 studies. However, the improvement in mortality was slight – between 4% and 6% among the studies.

The problem with this small result is that the studies these results came from were primarily of very elderly persons living in elderly-care facilities. This is problematic because they were undoubtedly deficient in vitamin D. And curiously, lower levels of vitamin supplementation – below 800 IU per day – did not change the risk of mortality. This brings into question dose-dependency, and the entire association of supplemented vitamin D.

It also brings into question whether vitamin D supplementation for a person who does get some sunlight will have the same effect if any.

The other problem with this result is that most of the patients given vitamin D in these studies were also given calcium supplements – because the two were taken together to help prevent osteoporosis. While a couple of different reviews found no difference between the effects of vitamin D with or without calcium, the calcium serves as a confounder – according to the researchers – especially when combined with the fact that the vitamin D dose did not make any difference.

The bottom line is that while unsulfated-vitamin D3 supplementation might indeed provide some help to those severely deficient in blood vitamin D levels, it remains to uncertain whether vitamin D supplementation by those who get even a marginal amount of sunlight exposure is even therapeutic.

The understanding of whether supplemented unsulfated-D3 is therapeutic may not be factually determined until at least researchers begin measuring and differentiating between the different types of 25(OH)D within the bloodstream. Measuring calcitriol would be even better. Until this is done, the issue of whether even vitamin D3 supplementation is therapeutic at all will remain unresolved.

Otherwise we are simply connecting dots in the dark rather than establishing sheer relationships between supplementation and disease prevention.

This was underscored by two medical professors from the Wisconsin School of Medicine, who stated in their review of research:

"Efforts to standardize vitamin D measurement and improve understanding of the physiologic consequences of other vitamin D metabolites such as 3-epi and 24,25(OH)2D (and potentially other vitamin D compounds) are needed. Currently, measurement of circulating 25(OH)D is accepted as the approach to define an individual's vitamin D status. However, existing 25(OH)D assays may include other vitamin D metabolites such as the 3-epimer of 25(OH)D and 24,25(OH)2D. It seems unlikely that the controversy will soon be resolved."

What is known for certain is that the form of vitamin D our own bodies make when exposed to UVB sunlight is therapeutic, and our bodies need it.

Our SAD Indoor World

About ninety percent of humans in modern society now work indoors. One hundred years ago, this statistic was reversed. At least ninety percent if not more, of humans lived and worked outside or in locations where natural light was directly present. While there are many warnings present in the medical literature to stay away from the sun, the National Institutes of Mental Health in Bethesda, Maryland included the following statement in a 1988 report (Skwerer *et al.*) on seasonal affective disorder: *"Along with food, air and water, sunlight is the most important survival factor in human life."*

While millions of people have been diagnosed with **seasonal affective disorder** (or SAD) over the past few years, some estimate a good 25 million Americans are afflicted with some form of the disorder – at least the milder yet more pervasive **winter blues** version of SAD. According to Norman Rosenthal, M.D., who led the above study and has published many scientific papers on seasonal affective disorder and the necessity of sunlight to mental health, about 6% of Americans have SAD and 14% have winter blues. For some, a move from the southern latitudes to the northern latitudes precipitates the disorder. For some, **depression** seems to be associated. In nearly all cases, a lack of sunlight is present.

As the fall and winter descend upon those in northern or southern latitudes, sunlight hours decrease and melatonin levels should increase along with levels of dopamine and GABA. These three biochemicals work together to not only sedate and relax our bodies so we are more prepared to sleep and spend less time outside: They also work to boost our moods at the same time. Dopamine and GABA are both mood-boosters that balance the increase in melatonin to relax us during the winter months. However, poor diets, a lack of exercise, increased stress and a lack of natural light all counteract these mood biochemicals. Stress alone can boost cortisol and adrenaline, which make us more irritable and less relaxed. Stress and a poor diet, together with a reduction of light and exercise, toss our body cycles out the window. We are now subject to a wicked combination of stress chemicals and imbalanced hormones. The result is the millions of SAD cases throughout our modern society.

SAD becomes a vicious cycle. As our stressload increases and our sunlight decreases, our hormones and other biochemicals go out of whack. Most people will try to resolve the issue with more activity indoors, most of which increases our stressload. As stressload increases, SAD symptoms increase.

A number of other diseases often comingle with SAD and winter blues: **Hypertension, atherosclerosis, early dementia, Alzheimer's, multiple sclerosis, allergies, psoriasis, fibromyalgia, depression, arthritis,** and **low back pain** are only a few of the ailments linked to a lack of sun exposure. A lack of natural sunlight during the winter depresses the immune system, weakens **eyesight**, and lowers **endocrine activity** – disrupting hormone secretion. This lowers **concentration**, increases **stress** and contributes to **depression**. Studies have also shown that winter sunlight reduction increases **hyperactivity** in children.

Illustrating this, one of the fastest growing illnesses in modern society is **autoimmune disease.** Research from Australian National University (Staples *et al.* 2003) found a strong relationship between various autoimmune diseases and ultraviolet radiation exposure. One of the most prominent results of the study was evident among **multiple sclerosis, rheumatoid arthritis** and **insulin-dependent diabetes mellitus.** The research also analyzed photo-immunology trials that showed that UV-B radiation seems to reduce the Th1 cell-mediation process, which stimulates **inflammatory responses**. This new perspective was considered a factor additional to the metabolic effects of vitamin D production in the body (Ponsonby *et* *al.* 2002). Another report from Pennsylvania State University two years later confirmed this correlation.

In the converse, an increasing amount of research is indicating that a lack of sunshine during the day combined with the lack of complete darkness during the night – as our environment has become increasingly lit up at night – reduces melatonin availability. This reduction in melatonin has been linked with various types of cancers, including **breast cancer, prostate cancer, colorectal cancer** and **endometrial cancer** (Reiter *et al.* 2007).

In a study done by the Heschong Mahone Group (1999), students learning within environments with the most natural sunlight tested better and exhibited faster rates of **learning.** Another study supporting this was conducted earlier by Anderson *et al.* (1991).

University of Alabama researchers studied 16,800 adults over the age of 45. Higher levels of sunlight exposure increased **cognitive function.** The benefit was even greater among **depressed or near-depressed** adults (Kent *et al.* 2009).

It must be concluded that vitamin D supplementation is not necessarily the solution to SAD and winter blues. As we discussed in detail on pages 113-114, natural light is the significant issue in mood disorders. This was confirmed in the large study showing that SAD prevalence is less in Iceland – where there is less vitamin D production yet people go outdoors more in the winter – than on the East Coast of the U.S.

While vitamin D alone will certainly help, even northern sun provides many more benefits that can be put into a pill. These include, as we have discussed, the sun's thermal benefits, natural light benefits, color benefits and biomagnetic benefits. These stimulate the production of important mood hormones including serotonin, dopamine, GABA and melatonin – and reduce the body's stressload as illustrated previously.

Cancer and the Sun

But doesn't the sun cause cancer? Actually, in the decades following Dr. Palm's reports that children from sunny areas did not contract rickets, doctors have slowly taken notice that those with more sun exposure had lower rates of a variety of cancers.

In 1970, cancer mortality maps revealed that sunnier regions had lower mortality rates from **internal cancers** than did areas with lower sunlight. In 1980, Johns Hopkins University's Dr. Frank Garland reported an unmistakable distribution gradient attributing sunnier locations to lower mortality rates for **colon cancer** – the leading fatal cancer. This prompted Dr. Edward Gorham and associates to study the association between serum vitamin D levels and colon cancer. These studies also showed a strong correlation between colon cancer and reduced vitamin D levels. This prompted a flurry of new studies correlating vitamin D with cancers of various types (Mohr 2009).

In a review of cancer studies from 1970 to 1994, the American Cancer Society's journal, *Cancer* (Grant, 2002) reported that UV-B solar radiation is associated with a reduction of **cancers of the breast, colon, ovaries, prostate, bladder, kidney, lung, pancreas, rectum, stomach, uterus, and esophagus.** Dr. William Grant, the author of the research, noted that the reduction of some cancers ranged from 30-50% with adequate UV-B sun exposure.

Clinical studies have also indicated a 20-30% increase in **breast cancer** incidence, and a 10-20% increased fatality rate for breast cancer among vitamin D-deficient women (Nielsen 2007).

In August of 2007, Dr. Cedric Garland and fellow cancer researchers at the Moores Cancer Center/University of California determined through analysis that about 250,000 **colorectal cancer** cases and 350,000 **breast cancer** cases worldwide could be prevented with increased vitamin D from sunbathing. It was estimated that a quarter of these cases – 150,000 – could be prevented in the United States alone.

In 2006, Dr. Francis Boscoe and Dr. Maria Schymura from the University of New York at Albany's School of Public Health published a major study that confirmed that ultraviolet sun exposure lowers the risk of many types of cancer. Dr.s Boscoe and Schymura looked at over three million cancer cases that occurred between 1998 and 2002, and three million deaths from cancer between 1993 and 2002 in the United States. Patient information was cross-referenced with UV-B levels taken from satellite data in thirty-two regions of the U.S. Low UV-B exposure correlated with greater incidence and more deaths from **bladder cancer, Hodgkin's lym-**

phoma, myeloma, biliary cancer, prostate cancer, rectal cancer, stomach cancer, uterine cancer, vulva cancer, breast cancer, kidney cancer, leukemia, non-Hodgkin's lymphoma, pancreatic cancer, gallbladder cancer, and thyroid cancer.

Interestingly, **skin cancer** rates have gone up dramatically over the past four decades, at close to the same rates as other cancers have gone up. Does this mean more people have gone out into the sun? While some researchers propose that a suntanning trend began in the 1960s, if we consider this issue in relation to the industrial revolution, over the past century more people are working and living indoors than ever before in history. Hence, the assumption that people have been receiving more sun is perhaps an oversimplification.

In a study done in Australia of 1,014 subjects (Holman *et al.* 1986), there was no relationship between **melanoma** and sun exposure, with the exception of the rare **Hutchinson's melanoma.**

Research has confirmed lower melanoma rates among dark skinned populations, but they do get skin cancer – despite the fact that few dark-skinned people sunbathe. The increased level of melanin in dark-skinned people's epidermal layers screens or filters more ultraviolet radiation, decreasing skin exposure.

Furthermore, recent research has confirmed that cancer rates have continued to rise over the past two decades despite a dramatic rise in the use of sun-protective agents like sunscreen and hats; and decreased sunbathing in general. Research has also shown that modern society's awareness of the need for sun protection is at an all-time high. In one study (Stoebner-Delbarre 2005) of 33,021 French adults, 92% understood the sun increased the risk of skin aging and 89% understood it increased cancer risk. With few alternatives, the study's researchers concluded the continued increases in skin cancer are due to this awareness not translating into action. The other possibility might be that the sun doesn't cause cancer.

There are two basic types of skin cancer: **Melanoma** and **non-melanoma skin cancer.** Melanoma grows from dysfunctional melanocytes. Melanoma is the more dangerous of the two, rendering far lower survival rates compared to non-melanoma skin cancer. Yet true melanoma is also rarer. By far, most of the skin cancers diagnosed – at least in the United States – are non-melanoma-related. According to the American Cancer Society, about 62,190 new melanomas were diagnosed in the U.S. and over one million non-melanoma skin cancers were diagnosed in 2006. The Cancer Society also estimates 10,710 skin cancer deaths occurred in 2006 – with 7,910 of those being melanoma.

There are three basic types of cells in the epidermis layer: the *melanocytes,* the *squamous keratinocytes* and the *basal keratinocytes.* Melanoma is associated with genetic damage occurring in melanocytes, and non-melanoma is associated primarily with genetic damage in the keratinocytes. Non-melanoma is divided into two types; **basal cell carcinoma** and **squamous cell carcinoma.** Both of these non-melanoma types are considered *benign,* however. They both can spread if conditions are right, but in most cases, the spread is either slow or visually obvious. Melanoma is known to spread more quickly, leading to greater fatality rates. It can also easily be excised and stopped if caught early.

Basal cell carcinoma occurs at the deeper basal cell level. A good 70-90% of skin cancer is the basal cell version. As for the squamous cell type, this typically occurs around the face, lips, neck, or ears – yet also interestingly in the genital areas. These may form from **actinic keratoses** – which some refer to as sunspots. There are a number of other non-melanoma skin cancer types such as **Kaposi sarcoma** and **Merkel cell carcinoma,** but these are rare.

The precise mechanisms for both melanoma and non-melanoma skin cancers are still being debated. It is thought that ultraviolet-B rays penetrate the basal cells deep in the epidermis layer, creating genetic damage. Research however, has indicated a more complex multi-step scenario. Both the sun's ultraviolet-B (280-315 nanometers) and ultraviolet-A (315-400 nm) rays, especially intense during the mid-day, can produce *reactive oxygen species* (also called *free radicals*) among the tissues in the epidermis. These reactive oxygen species appear to induce genetic mutations among the DNA in the cells – *if they are not neutralized.* Should these free radicals not be neutralized by the body's protective mechanisms, then DNA damage may occur amongst the kerotinocyte skin cells. Research presented by the Sydney Cancer Center's Melanoma and Skin Cancer Research Institute at the *Photocarcinogenesis Symposium of the 14th International Congress on Photobiology* (Halliday *et al.* 2005)

showed that ultraviolet-A causes a similar amount of gene mutations as does ultraviolet-B. While ultraviolet-B mutations
predominated in the upper tumor areas, ultraviolet-A damage predominated at the basal (lower) layers.

But while research has resolved that these ultraviolet rays can
create mutagenesis – damaging DNA – the picture is still more
complex, as there appears to be a decreased presence of mutation-
suppressors and mutation-repair mechanisms available among ultra-
violet-damaged tumors (Nishigori *et al.* 2004). Again, we find other
factors evident besides simply the impact of ultraviolet radiation
onto the skin.

Melanoma has been the fastest growing cancer in America
(Fecher 2007). While it was assumed that sun exposure was the
causal agent in non-Hodgkin types of melanoma, three recent studies have revealed that risk for melanoma actually decreased from
25% to 40% with increased recreational sun exposure. One study
(Armstrong 2007) indicated that possibly this effect is related to
higher-levels of vitamin D intake.

Recent studies are now illustrating that vitamin D reduces a
wide variety of cancers, including **prostate, colon** and **breast cancer** (Schwartz 2007). The connection between sun exposure and
skin cancer has thus been connected to immunosuppression – deficiencies of the body's immune system and antioxidant levels to
regulate and neutralize oxidization and the free radicals that cause
damage within the tissues (de Vries *et al.* 2007).

Research at the National Cancer Institute of the National Institutes of Health (Millen, *et al.* 2004) studied 1,607 outpatients from
various clinics, including 502 newly diagnosed **melanoma** patients.
Their diets were studied in detail. Those with diets low in alpha-
carotene, beta-carotene, cryptoxanthin, lutein and lycopene – all
plant-based food nutrients – had significantly higher levels of risk
of melanoma. Alcohol consumption was also significantly associated with higher risk of melanoma. And of course, lower vitamin D
levels were also associated with higher melanoma incidence in this
study. This means that eating a good diet of plant-based foods,
along with lower alcohol intake and more sunshine decreases ones
risk of melanoma.

Other studies have confirmed the link between diet and skin cancer. During the 1980s, several animal studies illustrated that UV-skin cancer occurred more readily with higher dietary fat intake. Switching back to a low-fat diet following UV-radiation dosing reversed the increased risk. In human research a few years later, 115 **actinic keratosis** and **non-melanoma cancer** patients adopted diets of either 20% fat or 40% fat content for two years. Those with the lower fat content had significantly lower levels of keratosis, and significantly fewer cancer lesions (Black 1998).

Other research has indicated that certain types of dietary fats increase the risk of skin cancer. A 2005 study (Harris *et al.* 2005) of 656 people, including 335 **squamous cell carcinoma** patients at the Arizona Cancer Center reported on the link between fatty acids and cancer risk. Fourteen different fatty acids were studied and measured from red blood cells. It was determined that increased levels of *arachidonic acid* – a fatty acid prominent in most meats and saturated oils – increased the risk of skin cancer, and palmitic acid and palmtoleic acid decreased the risk of skin cancer. Palmitic acid is a saturated fat found in palm oils and dairy products, while palmtoleic acid is a monounsaturated fat found in nuts and certain plant foods. Arachidonic acid is also linked to increased risk of inflammation and autoimmune disorders.

Cooked (especially fried) meats also produce carcinogenic cyclic amines. In 2007, researchers (Mohr *et al.*) at the University of California at San Diego reviewed skin cancer research from 107 countries. **They found that skin cancer incidence was associated with lower levels of UV-B rays, obesity, and animal diets.**

The Department of Radiation Genetics at the Kyoto University in Japan (Matsumura *et al.* 1996) studied 32 cases of **basal cell carcinomas** among Japanese patients – 16 of which were developed in sun-exposed areas and 16 developed in less-exposed areas. In both groups (consistent many other studies) the p53 gene was seen as the primary site of mutation. Furthermore, 75% of the non-exposed group showed transversions – the exchange of nucleotides between purines and pyrimidines. This exchange of bases at the genetic level relates to the bonds making up the DNA molecule – creating a switching out between two different sequence types. Once again, the study's authors noted these results indicate a more complex mechanism other than simply sun exposure for skin cancer.

Transversions have been observed *in vitro* primarily within two mechanisms: From the impact of toxic molecules – including free oxygen species and various toxins like benzene – and from the impact of ionizing radiation. Ionizing radiation occurs from various electromagnetic sources such as microwaves and various electronic appliances. While the sun might be considered a potential source of ionizing radiation, a molecular environment capable of creating ions at an intensity of radiation causing that ionizing must exist within the mechanism. More importantly, an environment within the body must exist where those ions – or reactive species – remain un-neutralized.

While a popular myth has spread that all free radicals are damaging at any level, recent research is revealing that exposure to reasonable amounts of free radicals, or oxidative species, is necessary for sustained health. In a study performed at the University of Jena in Germany (Schultz *et al.* 2007), free radicals formed in the cell through glucose inhibition significantly extended lifespan. The effect was apparently because the immune system developed a resistance to the oxidative stress caused by the reactive oxidative species. Consistent with other observations of immune strengthening due to increased resistance, it appears that some free radical exposure is required by the body and its cells.

Yet we also know that an overexposure to free radicals is unhealthy and even carcinogenic. The question is where is the line between a healthy amount of free radicals and overexposure? As the above study illustrates, nature has a design for maintaining a healthy balance between antioxidants and free radicals. This assumption also provides the basis for understanding why skin cancers (and so many other cancers and autoimmune disorders) are largely diseases of the modern industrialized societies, where sunlight and other natural inputs have been replaced by synthetic and often toxic versions.

We might closely consider the mutagenic effects that ultraviolet-B radiation has upon plants. (Yes, plant genes can also damaged by ultraviolet-B radiation, causing lesions.) Healthy plants have natural protective and neutralizing mechanisms and phytochemicals that mitigate this genetic damage. This becomes evident when we see some plants remaining green and healthy even as they sit in the intense sun all day long. Other plants – even of the same species – that are poorly watered and/or poorly fertilized, will turn brown in the mid-day sun. On the cellular level, this browning effect would be comparable to the sun's exposure among poorly nourished human skin cells (Zaets *et al.* 2006).

This reality can be hard to swallow given the linear aspect of the sun-skin cancer link. In a recent review of numerous skin cancer studies by researchers from the University of Southern California's Keck School of Medicine, the researchers admitted, *"...controversy exists, especially in the use of sunscreens."* (Ivry *et al.* 2006)

Dangerous Sun Lotions

In addition to the dietary associations mentioned earlier, one important consideration for the dramatic increase in skin cancer among our generation is the impact upon the body by sunscreens and other chemicals we spread onto our skin. Many of the chemical ingredients in many sunscreens have been identified as carcinogenic. These include benzophenone-3, homosalate, 4-methyl-benzylidene camphor, octylmethoxycinnamate, and octyl-dimethyl-PABA. These five, alone or in some combination thereof, are contained in about 90% of today's commercial sunscreens. All five have showed increased cancer cell proliferation both *in vitro* and *in vivo* in a study conducted at the Institute of Pharmacology and Toxicology at the University of Zurich (Schlumpf *et al.* 2001). This study also showed negative estrogenic and endocrine effects among mice from several of these chemicals.

A study done at the University of Manitoba in Winnipeg (Sarveiya *et al.* 2004) reported that all sunscreen ingredients tested – including octymethoxycinnamate and oxybenzone – significantly penetrate the skin. The penetration of common sunscreens was found to increase the penetration of even more dangerous herbicides – a concern for agricultural workers and non-organic gardeners (Pont *et al.* 2004). Furthermore, it has been established that some organic sunscreens can cause **photo-contact allergies** (Maier and Korting 2005). Research from Australia's Skin and Cancer Foundation (Cook and Freeman 2001) reported 21 cases of

photo-allergic contact dermatitis caused by oxybenzone, butyl methoxy dibenzoylmethane, methoxycinnamate or benzophenone. The Cook and Freeman research has led to a conclusion that these sunscreen ingredients are the leading cause of photo-allergic contact dermatitis.

Contact dermatitis is actually quite rare amongst the general population. A study at the National Institute of Dermatology in Colombia conducted a study of eighty-two patients with clinical photo-allergic contact dermatitis. Their testing showed that twenty-six of those patients – 31.7% – were shown to be positive for sensitivity to one or several of the sunscreen ingredients (Rodriguez *et al.* 2006).

The widespread proliferation of these harmful sunscreen ingredients – an occurrence increasing since the 1960s sunbathing era – is a significant factor in the skin cancer epidemic. Their addition to the epidermis layer create an environment of excessive oxidative radicals, as the sun in the presence of oxygen further oxidizes these synthetic molecules without nature's balancing biomolecules. At the bare minimum, these chemicals substantially increase the toxic burden within skin cells. This burden minimizes the body's ability to neutralize the oxidizing effects of the sun's radiation – intensifying the oxidizing factor. This intensification would essentially convert the sun's rays from therapeutic to dangerous.

Prior and concurrent to the prevalent use of sunscreen, sun-worshipers have ceremoniously applied various chemical- and oil-based sun lotions onto the skin. This is done to intensify the sun's tanning effects: to obtain that rich, brown tan to look more attractive. Many chemicals are/were in these products, including various hydrocarbons, which revert to oxidized radicals when exposed to the sun. In addition to sun lotion, sunbathers also apply various other chemical-based lotions onto the skin to condition, hydrate or treat sunburn. These various moisturizing lotions also contain a variety of synthetic chemicals that can become free radicals.

Furthermore, many sunscreens available today effectively absorb UV-B rays, but let UV-A rays through. Because UV-A rays are quite dangerous out of balance with UV-B to an unhealthy body, the risk of skin cancer using these sunscreens is even higher than without any sunscreen protection. In a 2007 study from the University of California at San Diego, researchers (Gorham *et al.* 2007) reviewed 17 studies of sunscreen use and melanoma. For those studies performed in latitudes over 40 degrees from the equator where skin types are fairer, there was a more significant correlation between sunscreen use and skin cancer.

Sun Dosage

The amount of sun dosage depends upon the melanin content of our skin. The darker our body is, the less exposure our melanocytes have to UVB rays, and the less vitamin D our body will produce. At the same time, darker skin will allow more time in the sun without burning, so it can balance out.

We know now with certainty that the active and most therapeutic version of vitamin D is 1,25-dihydroxyvitamin D_3 produced through the conversion of sunlight. It is also thought that the availability of 1,25-dihydroxyvitamin D in the tissues and bloodstream is raised – and possibly somewhat regulated – by the levels of isoflavones in the body. Isoflavones are nutrients available in various plant foods, with higher levels in grains and beans (Wietrzyk 2007).

Not many foods contain vitamin D. It is found in various dairy products such as cheese, butter, and cream, and in some fish and oysters, but the sun or supplements are the most reliable sources. The average American diet will only provide about 100-300 IU at the most. Dr. Grant reports that 2,000 to 4,000 IU is required for significant cancer rate reduction (i.e., with a poor diet).

Researchers at University of California (Garland *et al.* 2007) estimated that vitamin D levels of 52 nanograms per milliliter of serum (ng/ml) (equivalent to 4000 IU dosage) had 50% less risk of breast cancer than those with less than 13 ng/ml per day (equivalent to 1000 IU dosage). Minimally protective benefits were seen at 24 ng/ml (1845 IU dosage).

Leading vitamin D researcher Dr. Michael Holick recommends maintaining serum levels of no less than 20 ng/ml. This is equivalent to approximately a 1530 IU dose per day. Others have suggested that anything below 50 ng/ml is insufficient or deficient, while anything greater than 100 ng/ml is maximal.

Sunlight exposure at over 2500 lux with UV-B radiation produces sufficient vitamin D through the summer and parts of the spring and fall through most of the United States. This is less for northern states. Just twelve to twenty minutes of sunlight on the arms, legs, hands and face – with the sun at a 45-degree angle or more – will produce from 400 IU to 1000 IU of vitamin D for the average skin type, depending upon the health and metabolism of the person. A few hours of summer sun in a bathing suit until the skin is pink (not advisable) can produce as much as 20,000 IU. A day in the tropics could easily result in 100,000 IU/day. Although the RDA is 200-700 IU (700 for elderly adults), many nutritionists believe that 1,000 to 4,000 IU per day is optimal.

Exposure to enough sun to produce vitamin D is insufficient above latitude 42 degrees north (Azimuth) for six months of the year (November through February) (Cranney *et al.* 2007). This is about at the northern border of California on the west coast and Boston on the east coast. Below latitude 34 north, sun exposure is enough for year-round vitamin D production (Holick 2006). Between latitudes 34 and 42, the exposure is proportional. For northern latitudes, summertime vitamin D production generally takes place between about 11 a.m. and 1 p.m. Using the 45-degree sun angle is a good approximation. If your shadow is shorter than you, you are probably able to make vitamin D.

Cloud cover can reduce vitamin D production by about 50%, and smog can reduce it as much as 60% (Wharton *et al.* 2003). Vitamin D production does not occur from sun shining through a window, because UV-B does not penetrate glass (Holick 2005).

Therefore, some have suggested that it is better to be above the 50 degree north Azimuth, given city atmospheric conditions, clouds or haze. To look up your local Azimuth given a particular date, link to: http://aa.usno.navy.mil/data/docs/AltAz.php. Put in the date to test, state and nearest city. A chart will be produced. Look up the times where the Azimuth is above 45 degrees for clear, sunny weather, or 50 degrees during cloudy or hazy weather. The times will suggest the periods we can expose our skin to receive the maximal UV-B exposure and vitamin D production.

There has been some recent debate whether vitamin D is produced inside the epidermis or on top of the skin, within the sebum (fat) produced within the epidermis. While vitamin D3 can be obtained from the lanolin and fat within the skin of sheep – often used to make vitamin D supplements – this does not mean that vitamin D is produced on the skin. As shown by Dr. Hollick's research, vitamin D3 is produced within the epidermis, as the sebum was removed from the skin surface in these experiments. This should illustrate the production within the skin.

As the conjecture goes, some of that vitamin D3 may still remain on top of the dermis (skin surface) requiring a day or two to fully be absorbed into the skin. The conjecture thus suggests not showering or soaping off in order to conserve the vitamin D3.

It must be emphasized that there is no evidence to indicate this. Still, it may be possible that some of the vitamin D3 produced in the epidermal region may indeed be secreted to the surface, along with sebum and other waste as the body cleanses itself of toxins through the skin.

But refraining from cleaning the skin for two days would allow the potential of bacteria build up on the skin. Yes, the skin produces its own mucosal membrane that can control these colonies. But one sniff of skin that has been unwashed for two days will reveal unhealthy bacteria buildup.

One argument made to the hypothesis is that Hawaiian surfers tend to have lower vitamin D levels than lifeguards, and this is supposedly proving that the water is washing off the vitamin D. This, however, is a weak assumption, because Hawaiian surfers receive less sun exposure than lifeguards due to their legs being under water while they wait for waves.

This assumption that vitamin D is produced on top of the skin also contradicts the repeated research showing significantly high blood vitamin D levels are produced with sun exposure. None required the participants to avoid showering for two days.

The bottom line is that we know from direct evidence that vitamin D is produced within the epidermis. And yes, some may be secreted onto the skin with sebum. That means we may wash off some of the vitamin D. But this in no way discounts that we can produce and absorb healthy levels and still take a shower.

The more concerning issue is sunscreen. Sunscreen is robbing us of our necessary vitamin D, and the other tremendous benefits of the sun. An SPF-8 sunscreen will block about 95% of vitamin D synthesis, while possibly not even blocking damaging UV-A rays (Wolpowitz and Gilchrest 2006).

This later point brings up another speculative discourse, and that is that morning sun and evening sun will produce a higher risk of cancer because they contain more UV-A rays and fewer UV-B rays. This again, is speculative. The fact is, when the sun is lower in the sky, more UV-A and UV-B levels are being blocked. This is why it is less bright during these hours of the day. It is still important to receive sunlight during these hours of the day because of the effect that light in general has upon our pineal glands, and our production of melatonin and other important hormones.

This doesn't mean that we overdo it either. Getting sun in the early morning and late evening does little for our vitamin D levels, but these times are important for our exposure to the sun for other reasons, as we've discussed extensively in this book.

This brings us to the possibility that tanning beds offer a solution for vitamin D deficiency. To some degree, they might. A 2008 Boston University Medical School study noted that tanning beds produce therapeutic levels of 1,25-dihydroxyvitamin D_3. However, studies have also reported higher incidence of melanoma among tanning bed users. In one study of 551 persons, those who used tanning beds more than 20 minutes per session had significantly higher rates of malignant melanoma (Ting *et al.* 2007).

One of the issues to consider with tanning beds is that the UV-A/UV-B proportion can be extremely high. This high proportion may allow increased exposure without visible burning, hiding skin damage. New suntanning beds have come out recently that produce a more balance of rays. These may be beneficial for increasing vitamin D production for high latitude winters. While they can increase our vitamin D levels, their use should accompany caution and research. Nonetheless, they will not replace the sun's rays in general, so even when using tanning beds, it is advisable to spend considerable time outside in the sun.

Hypervitaminosis-D (high vitamin D levels) can be a consideration for supplementation. Some research has illustrated liver or kidney issues and even bone loss might result from extremely high serum levels of vitamin D. This has led researchers to conclude that extreme vitamin D doses may cause toxicity. Vitamin D from sun exposure is ameliorated by melanin production – nature's sunscreen.

Caution should accompany going from no sun to a tropical location or summer and spending too much time in the sun too soon. The best scenario is to slowly graduate our exposure to the sun as our body produces more melanin. In other words, we gradually increase our sun exposure as we begin to tan.

Most of the benefits of the sun occur through the stratum corneum of the epidermis. This is the outer layer of the skin. Research has attempted to quantify the dose needed for health benefit – referred to as the *minimal erythema dose* (ME dose or MED). This minimal effective dose is considered the minimum dose required to produce a slight reddening of the skin. However, the amount of sun required to accomplish this dose is different for each skin type. A darker-skinned person, for example, will require several times the amount of sun than a fairer-skinned person might. A dark African American may require from ten or twenty times the amount of sunlight a Caucasian might to achieve the same vitamin D production. However, multiple studies have indicated that possibly, African Americans require slightly lower levels of vitamin D than Caucasians to maintain health.

There are six basic skin types. They range from the fairest skin type at number one to the darkest skin with the number six. While the number one skin type might quickly burn and require only about 10 minutes of mid-day summer sun to establish an ME dose, a number six skin type will take about four times longer or 40 minutes, with little chance of burning. Most Caucasian people fall into the number three skin type, which might require about 20-30 minutes before establishing the minimum dose level.

This minimal dose might even be too much for someone not accustomed to the sun – at least until some tolerance is developed. Sunlight studies from Russia have indicated that about 30% to 60% of the ME dose levels are advisable until this tolerance is built up among the skin cells. This tolerance comes from a build up of melanin in the skin cells as mentioned. Melanin effectively shields the skin from UV over-exposure. With gradual exposure, melanin levels rise. ME dose can increase with increased melanin.

When humans lived primarily out-of-doors, the build-up of melanin was typical, and naturally protected us from these longer waves throughout life. Occasional sunlight – such as vacation exposure – exposes skin without melanin protection. Melanin protects skin cells in other ways, preserving their (anti-cancer) folate content and protecting the cell from other radical damage.

In the beginning, a fair-skinned person (type 1-2) should receive about ten minutes of arm-leg-face overhead sun in the summer, or better yet, about 30-45 minutes in the early evening or mid-morning sun to achieve a therapeutic dose of sun (lat. 34-42 degrees). A medium-skinned person (type 2-4) with more melanin should get about 15 minutes of overhead sun or better 45-60 minutes of morning or early-evening sun in the beginning. This increases to 20 minutes overhead or 75 minutes early/late sun for darker-skinned people (type 3-5) and 30 minutes overhead sun and 90 minutes of early/late sun for darker skin types (5-7) each day to achieve ME.

It will take longer to achieve a therapeutic dose at latitudes north of 42, and these should be focused upon the middle of the day. During the wintertime, the focus should also be upon the mid-day for those who live south of latitude 42. For those who live north of latitude 42, wintertime will not deliver vitamin D production (exceptions at high altitudes). Spending time outside during the day is still critical for the other reasons mentioned in this book.

For those living north of latitude 42, vacationing in a tropical place a couple of times during the winter is a good idea for vitamin D production, because we do store vitamin D (research has indicated a month or more) long after a trip to the tropics. This, in addition to vitamin D_3 supplementation, is not a bad idea. Getting outside into whatever sun is available is necessary at any rate.

Healthy Skin Nutrition

Both UV-A and UV-B rays have been accused of harming the skin. While UV-B causes sunburn if exposed for too long, UV-A has been shown to damage epidermal cells and DNA without the protection of melanin. Most physicians and researchers believe this protection consists of covering the body with chemicals to shield out the sun completely. This is a poor strategy, of course, because without the sun we will not produce vitamin D. Nor will we achieve many of the other benefits of the sun discussed elsewhere in this book.

In addition, we are faced with beauty consultants who tell us that the sun's exposure will leave us with a condition called **photoaging.** Photoaging is the process where the skin becomes rough and dry, with increased wrinkling. While this development is seemingly linked to the dosage of sunlight, there are many other issues to consider.

Photoaging is thought to be primarily caused by UV-A damage to dermal cells. However, the real reason for aged dry and wrinkly skin is a loss of keratin, collagen and elastin from deep within the dermal layer. Elastin and keratin are extracellular matrix proteins produced in tissue cells. They work together to help tissue systems such as muscles, ligaments and organs regain their original structure and size after being stretched or otherwise stressed. They also help maintain flexibility among skin cells. Elastin and keratin are made up of amino acids such as proline, alanine, glycine, valine and others. Keratins also contain significant levels of cysteine, which contains sulfur – bioavailable from plant nutrients. Meanwhile, lysine is involved in a catalyst for the assembly of elastin. Collagen is a stronger and more fibrous type of protein. Collagen helps tissue systems such as bone, ligaments and tendons maintain structure. In the skin, collagen gives structure, and balances the flexibility rendered by elastin and keratin. There are well over two dozen types of collagen molecules in the body. Most of these also contain proline and glycine. Many collagens also require a lysine derivative step, and utilize vitamin C and other phytonutrients for their assembly.

The point of this discussion is that the skin's elasticity and youthfulness is directly related to nutrition and protein assembly. Yes, an abundance of free radicals can deplete or interrupt the production of collagens, elastins and keratins. Quite simply, nearly every process in the body can be interrupted by radical species. This is where antioxidants come in. This is also where glutathione – a powerful antioxidant produced by the liver derived from phytonutrients – comes in. The antioxidant elements provided by plant-based nutrients render protective processes that neutralize radical species, allowing the body to produce the proteins necessary for skin structure and elasticity.

In other words, the health of the skin is directly related to its nutritional inputs. This includes oxygen, minerals, vitamins, antioxidants, water and many others. Without the right nutritional inputs, the dermal cells lie unprotected to neutralize free radicals created from not just the sun, but from any environmental input. White skin cells might look healthier for a time, but this precious-looking white skin may also be hiding a malnourished condition within. Soft white skin also looks good on a corpse.

Some scoff at such a proposal – that nutrients will prevent the damaging effects of UV-A and UV-B exposure. This is only because they have not seen the studies, and have not thoroughly examined the evidence.

A growing database of research illustrates that certain nutrients prevent or delay sunburn caused by UV-B, and minimize any damaging effects of UV-A. In late 2007, researchers from the Munster University Medical Center (Köpcke and Krutmann 2008) reported in a meta-study that analyzed seven different human trials revealing that beta-carotene supplementation protected against sunburn and other skin damage. In these studies, significant protection was accomplished with at least 10 weeks of supplementation prior to the heightened exposure. This is *seven different studies,* on humans, performed by medical researchers, and published in peer-reviewed medical research publications.

In a further study of the protective effects of certain nutrients, Heinrich *et al.* (2003) gave 24 human volunteers either an algae supplement containing 24 milligrams of beta-carotene, 8 mg of lutein and 8 mg of lycopene per day; or a placebo. After twelve weeks, the algae-supplemented group of 12 people had significantly lower erythema (pinkness) after sun exposure. Furthermore, the supplemented group showed faster skin recovery 24 hours after exposure. This study was published in the prestigious *Journal of Nutrition.*

In 2001, the *Journal of Nutrition* (Stahl *et al.*) published another study, this one illustrating that eating tomato paste significantly reduced the risk of sunburn. Nineteen volunteers consumed either 40 grams of tomato paste (containing 16 mg/g lycopene) or a placebo for ten weeks. After the ten weeks, both groups were exposed to harsh UV-A and UV-B exposure. The tomato-paste group experienced an average of 40% less erythema than did the controls.

Many other phytonutrients have also been shown to help protect the body from ultraviolet skin damage and skin cancers. The Cedrangolo Medical College of Italy's Second University (D'Angelo *et al.* 2005) reported a study using human melanoma cell lines and UV-A radiation. The major antioxidant compound in olives – hydroxytyrosol – protected against oxidative stress and the cascade towards melanoma.

Astaxanthin, a phytonutrient within algae such as spirulina and *Haematococcus pluvialis,* has been shown to exert a significant and powerful protective effect against sunburn and UV-A damage. Astaxanthin has been the subject of a number of studies over the past decade, showing greater skin-damage protective effects than even beta-carotene (Guerin *et al.* 2003).

These and many other studies have shown these same effects with other phytonutrients (nutrients from plants). Consumption of tocopherols including vitamin E, ascorbates including vitamin C, plant flavonoids and plant sterols have all been shown to reduce the impact of sunburn and protect the skin against irradiation damage. The consensus of this research on the mechanism is that these micronutrients produce a combination of effects. They absorb ultraviolet radiation. They reduce free radicals through antioxidation. They also modulate UV exposure signaling pathways, which increases resistance to any exposure damage (Sies and Stahl 2004).

The research also illustrates that popping a few vitamins before going on vacation is not going to cut it. This might help of course, but the dramatic effects produced by these studies require long-term dietary changes. A little supplementation a few days before significant sun exposure will certainly have positive benefits, but not the significant effects noted here.

Nutrients that nourish and protect skin cells are available mostly from plant-based foods. These phytonutrients are most easily obtained from a well-rounded whole food plant-based diet. Some of the most important phytonutritional components include beta-carotene, flavonoids, zeaxanthin and lycopene from carrots, tomatoes, leafy greens, cucumbers, celery, squash and others; anthocyanins from oats, red berries and cherries; lignans found in various grains and beans; sterols from greens, nuts and beans; flavonoids from just about every plant-based food; and many others.

The lowly eggplant provides a good example of the corrective properties phytochemicals provide to the skin. Eggplants contain a class of phytochemicals called solasodine glycosides. One of these, called solamargine, binds to sugar receptors (endogenous endocytic lectins) inside of cancer cells. This molecular binding results in solamargine being drawn into the cell's lysosomes, causing the lysosome to rupture. This rupturing causes the death of the cancer cell (Lee *et al.* 2004). This is only one phytonutrient out of many that provides anticarcinogenic effects.

Imbalanced oil consumption or the over-consumption of trans-fats can create weak cell membranes. The stronger the bonds among our phospholipid-rich cell membranes, the more protection the cells will have against *lipoxidation* damage. A balance of omega-3 oils DHA (from DHA Algae), ALA (from walnuts, chia and flax), GLA (from spirulina, borage and primrose) and omega-6 oils (from nuts and seeds) can effectuate healthy cell membranes.

The phytonutrients from plants are designed for ultraviolet radiation protection. In fact, most of the same phytonutrients that help protect our cells from ultraviolet damage also happen to help protect plants from sun damage. Healthy plants can survive the sun all day long without ultraviolet damage because of the protection provided by phytochemicals such as beta-carotene, lycopene, lutein, zeaxanthin and others.

In a nutritionally deficient system, wavelengths of ultraviolet-B and ultraviolet-A rays damage cells weakened through reduced nutrient content and increased toxin content. Toxins such as plasticizers, formaldehyde, organophosphates, alkylphenols, inorganic arsenic, phthalates, polychlorinated biphenyls (PCBs), volatile and semi-volatile organic compounds all burden the immune system and weaken cells.

These toxins are all prevalent among our modern day population. In 2007, the Environmental Working Group's *Human Toxome Project* revealed some frightening statistics regarding the chemical poisoning of our bodies. In one study of nine typical adult participants, blood and urine samples contained 171 of the 214 toxic chemicals that were screened for – including many mentioned above. These toxic chemicals create a surplus of oxidative species throughout the body. They also suppress the immune system as our bodies work to purify the cells and tissues. Along with toxins and radical species, a suppressed immune system is one of the key markers for any type of cancer risk – including skin cancers.

A couple of toxins that are often overlooked when considering skin damage and skin cancer are smoking and alcohol. Many people drink and/or smoke during outings in the sun. Smoking does not just cause lung cancer: Cigarettes contain various toxins that burden the immune system, opening it up to skin and other cancers. Smoking also releases various free radicals into the body. Alcohol is also implicated in various cancers.

Alcohol also produces reactive oxygen species. Alcohol is a dehydrating agent to boot. Cells without enough hydration become stressed – and vulnerable to damage.

The strategy for keeping skin youthful and reducing the risk of skin cancer is to eat a predominantly plant-based diet containing significant antioxidant capacity; hydrate with plenty of water; exercise frequently to maintain good circulation; and get plenty of fresh air and sunlight.

Natural sunlight stimulates the production of hormones and neurotransmitters that encourage the repair of damage done by oxidative radicals. Natural sunlight warms the body with thermal radiation, stimulating the production of key enzymes that assist the immune system and its detoxification routines. Sunlight stimulates the production of vitamin D, one of the body's most critical nutrients. These combined mechanisms of the sun stimulate a stronger immune system – ready to balance free radicals while protecting the body's cells from radiation damage.

Even in a healthy body, numerous mutations occur on a daily basis. These form as the body deals with weakened cells and normal environmental stressors. A healthy immune system removes these as a matter of course before they have any chance to grow into larger tumors. An undernourished or burdened immune system, on the other hand, allows larger groups of cancer cells to grow from these mutations with little resistance.

Sunlight also stimulates the production of natural skin oils and melanin, which both provide further protection from any damage from the sun. An increase in the volume and activity of melanocytes assists the cells in the production of melanin. Melanin acts as a natural sunscreen mechanism, allowing the body to draw upon the sun's useful radiation with less oxidative damage. For this reason, traditional cultures with more sun exposure typically have browner skin. Cultures of colder climes became deficient in melanin after many generations. This is easily remedied, however. A gradual increase in sun exposure over a period of time will radically increase the skin cells' melanin levels in most skin types – reducing potential damage from ultraviolet oxidation.

Furthermore, as our bodies resonate with the sun's electromagnetic radiation, the destructive nature of anxiety and stress is reduced. A moderate amount of sunshine helps relax the nerves and stimulates the production of positive mood neurotransmitters such as serotonin, GABA and dopamine. Healthy sun also improves our sleep quality and quality of life in general.

Healthy Sunbathing Strategies

* **Creams and Sunscreen:** Sun exposure is best without any creams or lotions. Many lotions have toxic ingredients, as discussed. Even the healthiest oils and lotions can become oxidized or otherwise degraded by the sun's rays, creating free radicals and denatured molecules.

* **Semi-covered exposure:** We can start by taking walks, gardening or sitting outside while allowing the sun's rays to shine upon our heads, feet, arms, and hands. The areas of the body covered with hair, such as the arms, legs and top of the head should be exposed first.

* **Staged sunbathing:** Once ready for sunbathing, the fair-skinned should begin with a few minutes in the morning sun during the springtime. Expose skin in stages: First arms and legs. Then neck and shoulders. Then chest and back. Gradually build up melanin content on each area. This is confirmed by a light brown skin color. Skin type, previous sun exposure, time of day and location are determining factors for how much exposure is healthy. Gradually increase sun duration as the spring proceeds.

* **Avoid erythema:** In no case should the exposure result in a pink skin color. This is a sunburn regardless of the "burn."

* **Sun maturity:** This slow build-up should allow 1-2 hours in morning or late afternoon sun without burning.

* **Clouds:** Cloudy or sunny, we still receive the sun's wave-forms. The sun's UV-A and UV-B waves will penetrate cloud cover at about 50%. This means we can still produce vitamin D, and still sunburn on a cloudy day.

* **The face:** Because the face receives the greatest intermittent sun exposure and likely contains the most melanin, other areas will produce more vitamin D. The face is probably best covered during sunbathing. Visors are great because they allow the sun to hit the top of the head.

* **Store-up vitamin D:** Because vitamin D is stored in the fat cells, we can store up enough vitamin D to get us through a few rainy, colder days. If we are north of latitude 42, we can head south every so often (monthly will work) during the winter to replenish our vitamin D stores. Even north of latitude 42, getting out into the sun is still important for moods, energy, cognition and biomagnetism.

* **Vacation:** A vacation in the tropics, where the sun can be 5-10 times more intense, or an extended period outside can provide enough vitamin D for a month or more. It is still important to be outside for the sun's other benefits.

* **Sunbathing seasons:** Sunbathing with seasonal rhythm is essential. South of latitude 42 and north of latitude 34, the best time for winter sunbathing is in the mid-day. During the summer, late mornings and mid afternoons are best for vitamin D. South of latitude 34, mid-mornings and afternoons are best all year round. For areas north of latitude 42, mid-day sun is best all year round, though November and February will yield little vitamin D in these areas.

* **Underbelly vitamin D:** For the time-crunched, or during winter (south of latitude 42, north of latitude 34), exposing

underbelly parts can yield faster vitamin D production. 'Underbelly' parts: the armpits, backs of the arms, knees, feet, neck; and the belly and butt (assuming privacy). Remember, these areas will burn faster too, so shorter durations or weaker sun positions are required for these parts.

* **Hairy parts:** Hairy parts of the body are more protected than non-hairy parts, depending upon the hair color (darker color provides more protection). These areas can receive more sunbathing time, but be careful to avoid any pink.

* **Take extra clothes:** Even in summer, we should have long pants and long-sleeved shirts available to reduce exposure.

* **Sunbathing clothed:** We receive some of the sun's spectrum of healthy waveforms while clothed. These include radio, infrared and biomagnetic waves. These invigorate the nervous system, calm the mind and regulate hormones.

* **Window bathing:** For those who have trouble getting outside, the sun can be brought through the window. The window should be opened, however, to avoid an imbalance between UV-A and UV-B rays. Glass blocks the sun's UV-B radiation, so we cannot produce vitamin D next to a window. Sunbathing through glass should be used with extreme caution, as too much UV-A rays can produce cancer.

* **Reading and meeting outside:** Natural sunlight boosts cognition, and stimulates creativity. Learning ability increases in schoolrooms with more natural light or outdoor seating. Behavior and moods are more balanced and relaxed. Walks in the sun help us think things through. We find solutions easier, and can better get perspective. We can see the bigger picture – and prioritize things. Within a natural setting and under the sun's rays, we may understand just how unimportant our issues really are.

* **Healthy sun diet:** An antioxidant-rich diet and good hydration is critical to healthy sun exposure. A diet rich in colorful foods and fiber will curb free radical formation.

* **Healing with the sun:** Sun exposure stimulates the immune system and increases detoxification. With or without direct skin exposure, we can benefit. Check with personal health professional first, especially if taking any medications. Some medications can cause photosensitivity.

* **The healthiest sunscreens:** Hat, clothing, shade trees. Chemical sunscreens should be avoided, unless cover and clothes are not possible. If we must, we can choose "natural" versions, preferably without PABA and other chemicals mentioned earlier. Sunscreen lotions with zinc and added vitamins and botanicals can help neutralize free radicals, but they cannot replace dietary antioxidants.

* **Best sunburn remedy:** Burning should be avoided at all costs. If our bodies do get sun burnt, the best agent for relief and healing is *Aloe vera* gel. Natural aloe is easy to grow in any sunny environment. Aloe is used by breaking or cutting a small portion of leaf off the plant and peeling back its skin. We can rub the gel on skin. The juice of the aloe is not as bioactive as the gel. This milky plant's gel holds most of its effective constituents for the skin. Natural aloe gel contains aloectin, anthraquinones, polysaccharides, resins, and tannins. These phytochemicals work synergistically to speed healing, neutralize free radicals, and soothe pain.

* **Cucumber gel:** Also good for sunburn. Cucumber gel contains elaterin resin, starches, lignin, saline matter, and minerals. These help heal while providing antioxidants. Cooling fresh slices can be laid or rubbed over the skin, or crushed into a lotion.

* **Lemon:** Lemon is also helpful for sunburn. The combination of citric acid, citral, hesperidin sugars and limonenes give lemon a soothing and antioxidant effect upon the skin. Freshly squeezed lemons can be diluted in water 50/50 and sponged right onto the skin for immediate relief.

* **How to get skin cancer:** Eat lots of fried meats to increase our arachidonic acid and cyclic amine content. Eat

very few vegetables or fruits. Don't worry about eating foods with lots of pesticides, chemical preservatives and food dyes. Don't bother avoiding exposure to toxic chemicals. Slather on the PABA and octylmethoxycinnamate-based sunscreen lotions. Go out and immediately spend too much time in the sun. Drink alcohol and maybe even smoke while out in the sun. No worries about drinking enough water. Get sun burnt (after the sunscreen washes or sweats off), and then apply chemical-based skin lotions to cool and "moisturize" the skin.

References and Bibliography

Abdou AM, Higashiguchi S, Horie K, Kim M, Hatta H, Yokogoshi H. Relaxation and immunity enhancement effects of gamma-aminobutyric acid GABA. *Biofactors.* 2006;26(3):201-8.

Ackerman D. *A Natural History of the Senses.* New York: Vintage, 1991.

Ainsleigh HG. Beneficial effects of sun exposure on cancer mortality. *Prev Med.* 1992;22:132-40.

Airola P. *How to Get Well.* Phoenix, AZ: Health Plus, 1974.

Akbar-Khanzadeh F, Bitovski DK. Exposure of school employees to extremely low frequency magnetic fields. *Can J Public Health.* 2000 Jan-Feb;91(1):21-4.

Amassian VE, Cracco RQ, Maccabee PJ, Cracco JB, Rudell A, Eberle L. Suppression of visual perception by magnetic coil stimulation of human occipital cortex. *Electroencephalogr Clin Neurophysiol.* 1989 Nov-Dec;74(6):458-62.

Anderson DR, Huston AC, Schmitt KL, Linebarger DL, Wright JC. Early childhood television viewing and adolescent behavior: the recontact study. *Monogr Soc Res Child Dev.* 2001;66(1):I-VIII, 1-147.

Anderson MJ, Petros TV, Beckwith BE, Mitchell WW, Fritz S. Individual differences in the effect of time of day on long-term memory access. *Am J Psych.* 1991;104:241–255.

Apperley FL. The relation of solar radiation to cancer mortality in North America. *Cancer Res.* 1941;1:191-96.

Armas LA, Hollis BW, Heaney RP. Vitamin D2 is much less effective than vitamin D3 in humans. *J Clin Endocrinol Metab.* 2004 Nov;89(11):5387-91.

Armstrong B, Thériault G, Guénel P, Deadman J, Goldberg M, Héroux P. Association between exposure to pulsed electromagnetic fields and cancer in electric utility workers in Quebec, Canada, and France. *Am J Epidemiol.* 1994 Nov 1;140(9):805-20.

Armstrong BK, Kricker A. Sun exposure and non-Hodgkin lymphoma. *Cancer Epidemiol Biomarkers Prev.* 2007 Mar;16(3):396-400.

Aton SJ, Colwell CS, Harmar AJ, Waschek J, Herzog ED. Vasoactive intestinal polypeptide mediates circadian rhythmicity and synchrony in mammalian clock neurons. *Nat Neurosci.* 2005 Apr;8(4):476-83.

Autier P, Boniol M, Pizot C, Mullie P. Vitamin D status and ill health: A systematic review. Lancet Diab Endo. 2014; 2(1):76-89 doi:10.1016/S2213-8587(13)70165-7

Autier P, Gandini S, Mullie P. A systematic review: influence of vitamin D supplementation on serum 25-hydroxyvitamin D concentration. J Clin Endocrinol Metab. 2012 Aug;97(8):2606-13. doi: 10.1210/jc.2012.1238.

Autier P, Gandini S. Vitamin D supplementation and total mortality: a meta-analysis of randomized controlled trials. Arch Intern Med. 2007 Sep 10;167(16):1730-7.

Axelson M. 25-Hydroxyvitamin D3 3-sulphate is a major circulating form of vitamin D in man. FEBS Lett. 1985 Oct 28;191(2):171-5.

Azar JA, Conroy T. Measuring the effectiveness of horticultural therapy at a veterans administration medical center: experimental design issues. In Relf, D. (ed) *The Role of Horticulture in Human Well-Being and Social Development: A National Symposium.* Portland: Timber Press. 1992:169-171.

Backster C. *Primary Perception: Biocommunication with plants, living foods, and human cells.* Anza: White Rose, 2003.

Ballentine R. *Diet & Nutrition: A holistic approach.* Honesdale, PA: Himalayan Int., 1978.

Ballentine R. *Radical Healing.* New York: Harmony Books, 1999.

Baran D, Apostol I. Signification of biorhythms for human performance assessment. *Rev Med Chir Soc Med Nat Iasi.* 2007 Jan-Mar;111(1):295-302.

Barker A. *Scientific Method in Ptolemy's Harmonics.* Cambridge: Cambridge University Press, 2000.

Barone A, Giusti A, Pioli G, Girasole G, Razzano M, Pizzonia M, Palummeri E, Bianchi G. Secondary hyperparathyroidism due to hypovitaminosis D affects bone mineral density response to alendronate in elderly women with osteoporosis. *J Am Geriatr Soc.* 2007 May;55(5):752-7.

Barron M. Light exposure, melatonin secretion, and menstrual cycle parameters: an integrative review. Biol Res Nurs. 2007 Jul;9(1):49-69.

Becker R. *Cross Currents.* Los Angeles: Tarcher, 1990.

Becker R. *The Body Electric.* New York: Morrow, Inc., 1985.

Beecher GR. Phytonutrients' role in metabolism: effects on resistance to degenerative processes. *Nutr Rev.* 1999 Sep;57(9 Pt 2):S3-6.

Behin A, Hoang-Xuan K, Carpentier AF, Delattre JY. Primary brain tumours in adults. *Lancet.* 2003 Jan 25;361(9354):323-31.

Benedetti F, Radaelli D, Bernasconi A, Dallaspezia S, Falini A, Scotti G, Lorenzi C, Colombo C, Smeraldi E. Clock genes beyond the clock: CLOCK genotype biases neural correlates of moral valence decision in depressed patients. *Genes Brain Behav.* 2007 Mar 26.

Bennet LW, Cardone S, Jarczyk J. Effects of therapeutic camping program on addiction recovery. *Journal of Substance Abuse Treatment.* 1998;15(5):469-474.

Bensky D, Gable A, Kaptchuk T (transl.). *Chinese Herbal Medicine Materia Medica.* Seattle: Eastland Press, 1986.

Bentley E. *Awareness: Biorhythms, Sleep and Dreaming.* London: Routledge, 2000.

233

Berk M, Dodd S, Henry M. Do ambient electromagnetic fields affect behaviour? A demonstration of the relationship between geomagnetic storm activity and suicide. *Bioelectromagnetics.* 2006 Feb;27(2):151-5.

Berk M, Sanders KM, Pasco JA, Jacka FN, Williams LJ, Hayles AL, Dodd S. Vitamin D deficiency may play a role in depression. *Med Hypotheses.* 2007;69(6):1316-9.

Berman S, Fein G, Jewett D, Ashford F. Luminance-controlled pupil size affects Landolt C task performance. *J Illumin Engng Soc.* 1993;22:150-165.

Berman S, Jewett D, Fein G, Saika G, Ashford F. Photopic luminance does not always predict perceived room brightness. *Light Resch and Techn.* 1990;22:37-41.

Berry J. Work efficiency and mood states of electronic assembly workers exposed to full-spectrum and conventional fluorescent illumination. *Diss Abstr Internl.* 1983;44:635B.

Bertin G. *Spiral Structure in Galaxies: A Density Wave Theory.* Cambridge: MIT Press, 1996.

Besset A, Espa F, Dauvilliers Y, Billiard M, de Seze R. No effect on cognitive function from daily mobile phone use. *Bioelectromagnetics.* 2005 Feb;26(2):102-8.

Bhattacharjee C, Bradley P, Smith M, Scally A, Wilson B. Do animals bite more during a full moon? *BMJ.* 2000 December 23; 321(7276): 1559-1561.

Bickham DS, Rich M. Is television viewing associated with social isolation? Roles of exposure time, viewing context, and violent content. *Arch Pediatr Adolesc Med.* 2006 Apr;160(4):387-92.

Bierman DJ. Does Consciousness Collapse the Wave-Packet? *Mind and Matter.* 1993;1(1):45-57.

Binkley N, Wiebe D. Clinical controversies in vitamin D: 25(OH)D measurement, target concentration, and supplementation. J Clin Densitom. 2013 Oct-Dec;16(4):402-8. doi: 10.1016/j.jocd.2013.08.006.Grad B. A telekinetic effect on plant growth: II. Experiments involving treatment of saline in stoppered bottles. *Internl J Parapsychol.* 1964;6:473-478, 484-488.

Bishop ID, Rohrmann B. Subjective responses to simulated and real environments: a comparison. *Landscape and Urban Planning.* 2003;65(4):261-277.

Black HS. Influence of dietary factors on actinically-induced skin cancer. *Mut Res.* 1998 Nov 9;422(1):185-90.

Blackman CF, Benane SG, House DE, Pollock MM. Action of 50 Hz magnetic fields on neurite outgrowth in pheochromocytoma cells. *Bioelectromagnetics.* 1993;14(3):273-86.

Bodnar L, Simhan H. The prevalence of preterm birth varies by season of last menstrual period. *Am J Obst and Gyn.* 2003;195(6):S211-S211.

Bohay RN, Bencak J, Kavaliers M, Maclean D. A survey of magnetic fields in the dental operatory. *J Can Dent Assoc.* 1994 Sep;60(9):835-40.

Boivin DB, Czeisler CA. Resetting of circadian melatonin and cortisol rhythms in humans by ordinary room light. *Neuroreport.* 1998 Mar 30;9(5):779-82.

Boivin DB, Duffy JF, Kronauer RE, Czeisler CA. Dose-response relationships for resetting of human circadian clock by light. *Nature.* 1996 Feb 8;379(6565):540-2.

Bollani L, Dolci C, Gerola O, Montaruli A, Rondini G, Carandente F. The early maturation of the circadian system in newborns. *Chronobiologia.* 1994 Jan-Jun;21(1-2):105-8.

Boray P, Gifford R, Rosenblood L. Effects of warm white, cool white and full-spectrum fluorescent lighting on simple cognitive performance, mood and ratings of others. J Environl Psychol. 1989;9:297-308.

Boscoe FP, Schymura MJ. Solar ultraviolet-B exposure and cancer incidence and mortality in the United States, 1993-2002. BMC Cancer. 2006 Nov 10;6:264.

Boston University. Effects Of Vitamin D And Skin's Physiology Examined. ScienceDaily. 2008 February 24. Retrieved February 24, 2008, from http://www.sciencedaily.com/releases/2008/02/080220161707. htm. Accessed: 2008 Nov.

Boyce P, Rea M. A field evaluation of full-spectrum, polarized lighting. Paper presented at the 1993 Annual Convention of the Illuminating Engineering Society of North America, Houston, TX. 1993 Aug.

Boyce P. Investigations of the subjective balance between illuminance and lamp colour properties. *Light Resch and Technol.* 1977;9:11-24.

Brainard GC, Kavet R, Kheifets LI. The relationship between electromagnetic field and light exposures to melatonin and breast cancer risk: a review of the relevant literature. *J Pineal Res.* 1999 Mar;26(2):65-100.

Brenner D, Hall E. Computed Tomography – An Increasing Source of Radiation Exposure. *NE J Med.* 2007;357(22):2277-2284.

Breton ME, Montzka DP. Empiric limits of rod photocurrent component underlying a-wave response in the electroretinogram. *Doc Ophthalmol.* 1992;79(4):337-61.

Brodeur P. *Currents of Death.* New York: Simon and Schuster, 1989.

Brody J. *Jane Brody's Nutrition Book.* New York: WW Norton, 1981.

Brown FA, Chow CS. Lunar-Correlated variations in water uptake by bean seeds. *Biol B.* 1973 145:265-278.

Buckley NA, Whyte IM, Dawson AH. There are days ... and moons. Self-poisoning is not lunacy. *Med J Aust.* 1993 Dec 6-20;159(11-12):786-9.

Buijs RM, Scheer FA, Kreier F, Yi C, Bos N, Goncharuk VD, Kalsbeek A. Organization of circadian functions: interaction with the body. *Prog Brain Res.* 2006;153:341-60.

Bulsing PJ, Smeets MA, van den Hout MA. Positive Implicit Attitudes toward Odor Words. *Chem Senses.* 2007 May 7.

Burikov AA, Bereshpolova YuI. The activity of thalamus and cerebral cortex neurons in rabbits during "slow wave-spindle" EEG complexes. *Neurosci Behav Physiol.* 1999 Mar-Apr;29(2):143-9.

Buscemi N, Vandermeer B, Pandya R, Hooton N, Tjosvold L, Hartling L, Baker G, Vohra S, Klassen T. Melatonin for treatment of sleep disorders. *Evid Rep Technol Assess.* 2004 Nov;(108):1-7.

Buzsaki G. Theta rhythm of navigation: link between path integration and landmark navigation, episodic and semantic memory. *Hippocampus.* 2005;15(7):827-40.

Cahill RT. A New Light-Speed Anisotropy Experiment: Absolute Motion and Gravitational Waves Detected. *Progress in Physics.* 2006; (4).

Cai L, Mu LN, Lu H, Lu QY, You NC, Yu SZ, Le AD, Zhao J, Zhou XF, Marshall J, Heber D, Zhang ZF. Dietary selenium intake and genetic polymorphisms of the GSTP1 and p53 genes on the risk of esophageal squamous cell carcinoma. *Cancer Epidemiol Biomarkers Prev.* 2006 Feb;15(2):294-300.

Cajochen C, Jewett ME, Dijk DJ. Human circadian melatonin rhythm phase delay during a fixed sleep-wake schedule interspersed with nights of sleep deprivation. *J Pineal Res.* 2003 Oct;35(3):149-57.

Cajochen C, Zeitzer JM, Czeisler CA, Dijk DJ. Dose-response relationship for light intensity and ocular and electroencephalographic correlates of human alertness. *Behav Brain Res.* 2000 Oct;115(1):75-83.

Caldwell MM, Bornman JF, Ballare CL, Flint SD, Kulandaivelu G. Terrestrial ecosystems, increased solar ultraviolet radiation, and interactions with other climate change factors. *Photochem Photobiol Sci.* 2007 Mar;6(3):252-66.

Cantor KP, Stewart PA, Brinton LA, Dosemeci M. Occupational exposures and female breast cancer mortality in the United States. *J Occup Environ Med.* 1995 Mar;37(3):336-48.

Capitani D, Yethiraj A, Burnell EE. Memory effects across surfactant mesophases. *Langmuir.* 2007 Mar 13;23(6):3036-48.

Carlsen E, Olsson C, Petersen JH, Andersson AM, Skakkebaek NE. Diurnal rhythm in serum levels of inhibin B in normal men: relation to testicular steroids and gonadotropins. *J Clin Endocrinol Metab.* 1999 May;84(5):1664-9.

Celec P, Ostaniková D, Skoknová M, Hodosy J, Putz Z, Kúdela M. Salivary sex hormones during the menstrual cycle. *Endocr J.* 2009 Jun;56(3):521-3.

Celec P, Ostatníková D, Hodosy J, Putz Z, Kúdela M. Increased one week soybean consumption affects spatial abilities but not sex hormone status in men. *Int J Food Sci Nutr.* 2007 Sep;58(6):424-8.

Celec P, Ostatnikova D, Putz Z, Kudela M. The circalunar cycle of salivary testosterone and the visual-spatial performance. *Bratisl Lek Listy.* 2002;103(2):59-69.

Celec P. Analysis of rhythmic variance – ANORVA. A new simple method for detecting rhythms in biological time series. *Biol Res.* 2004;37(4 Suppl A):777-82.

Cengel YA, *Heat Transfer: A Practical Approach.* Boston: McGraw-Hill, 1998.

Cham, B. Solasodine glycosides as anti-cancer agents: Pre-clinical and Clinical studies. *Asia Pac J Pharmac.* 1994;9:113-118.

Chapman S, Morrell S. Barking mad? another lunatic hypothesis bites the dust. *BMJ.* 2000 Dec 23-30;321(7276):1561-3.

Chapman, S. Fear of frying: power lines and cancer. *BMJ* 2001;322:682.

Characterization and quantitation of Antioxidant Constituents of Sweet Pepper (Capsicum annuum - Cayenne). *J Agric Food Chem.* 2004 Jun 16;52(12):3861-9.

Chen-Goodspeed M, Cheng Chi Lee. Tumor suppression and circadian function. *J Biol Rhythms.* 2007 Aug;22(4):291-8.

Chirkova EN, Suslov LS, Avramenko MM, Krivoruchko GE. Monthly and daily biorhythms of amylase in the blood of healthy men and their relation with the rhythms in the external environment. *Lab Delo.* 1990;(4):40-4.

Chong NW, Codd V, Chan D, Samani NJ. Circadian clock genes cause activation of the human PAI-1 gene promoter with 4G/5G allelic preference. *FEBS Lett.* 2006 Aug 7;580(18):4469-72.

Cimetidine inhibits the hepatic hydroxylation of vitamin D. *Nutr Rev.* 1985;43:184-5.

Cochran ES, Vidale JE, Tanaka S. Earth tides can trigger shallow thrust fault earthquakes. *Science.* 2004 Nov 12;306(5699):1164-6.

Cocilovo A. Colored light therapy: overview of its history, theory, recent developments and clinical applications combined with acupuncture. *Am J Acupunct.* 1999;27(1-2):71-83.

Cohen S, Popp FA. Biophoton emission of the human body. *J Photochem Photobiol B.* 1997 Sep;40(2):187-9.

Coles JA, Yamane S. Effects of adapting lights on the time course of the receptor potential of the anuran retinal rod. *J Physiol.* 1975 May;247(1):189-207.

Collins RL, Elliott MN, Berry SH, Kanouse DE, Kunkel D, Hunter SB, Miu A. Watching sex on television predicts adolescent initiation of sexual behavior. *Pediatrics.* 2004 Sep;114(3):e280-9.

Contreras D, Steriade M. Cellular basis of EEG slow rhythms: a study of dynamic corticothalamic relationships. *J Neurosci.* 1995 Jan;15(1 Pt 2):604-22.

Cook N, Freeman S. Report of 19 cases of photoallergic contact dermatitis to sunscreens seen at the Skin and Cancer Foundation. *Australas J Dermatol.* 2001 Nov;42(4):257-9.

Cranney A, Horsley T, O'Donnell S, Weiler H, Puil L, Ooi D, Atkinson S, Ward L, Moher D, Hanley D, Fang M, Yazdi F, Garritty C, Sampson M, Barrowman N, Tsertsvadze A, Mamaladze V. Effectiveness and safety of vitamin D in relation to bone health. *Evid Rep Technol Assess.* 2007 Aug;(158):1-235.

Crawley J. *The Biorhythm Book.* Boston: Journey Editions, 1996.

Creinin MD, Keverline S, Meyn LA. How regular is regular? An analysis of menstrual cycle regularity. *Contraception.* 2004 Oct;70(4):289-92.

Crönlein T, Langguth B, Geisler P, Hajak G. Tinnitus and insomnia. *Prog Brain Res.* 2007;166:227-33.

Cuppari L, Garcia-Lopes MG. Hypovitaminosis D in chronic kidney disease patients: prevalence and treatment. *J Ren Nutr.* 2009 Jan;19(1):38-43.

Cutolo M, Straub RH. Circadian rhythms in arthritis: hormonal effects on the immune/inflammatory reaction. *Autoimmun Rev.* 2008 Jan;7(3):223-8.

D'Angelo S, Ingrosso D, Migliardi V, Sorrentino A, Donnarumma G, Baroni A, Masella L, Tufano MA, Zappia M, Galletti P. Hydroxytyrosol, a natural antioxidant from olive oil, prevents protein damage induced by long-wave ultraviolet radiation in melanoma cells. *Fr Rad Bio Med.* 2005 Apr 1;38(7):908-19.

Darby S, Hill D, Auvinen A, Barros-Dios JM, Baysson H, Bochicchio F, Doll R, *et al.* Radon in homes and risk of lung cancer: collaborative analysis of individual data from 13 European case-control studies. *BMJ.* 2005 Jan 29;330(7485):223.

Darby S, Hill D, Auvinen A, Bochicchio F, *et al.* Radon in homes and risk of lung cancer: collaborative analysis of individual data from 13 European case-control studies. *BMJ.* 2005 Jan 29;330(7485):223.

Davies G. *Timetables of Medicine.* New York: Black Dog & Leventhal, 2000.

Davis GE Jr, Lowell WE. Chaotic solar cycles modulate the incidence and severity of mental illness. *Med Hypotheses.* 2004;62(2):207-14.

Davis GE Jr, Lowell WE. Solar cycles and their relationship to human disease and adaptability. *Med Hypotheses.* 2006;67(3):447-61.

Davis GE Jr, Lowell WE. The Sun determines human longevity: teratogenic effects of chaotic solar radiation. *Med Hypotheses.* 2004;63(4):574-81.

Davis RL, Mostofi FK. Cluster of testicular cancer in police officers exposed to hand-held radar. *Am J Ind Med.* 1993 Aug;24(2):231-3.

Davis S, Kaune WT, Mirick DK, Chen C, Stevens RG. Residential magnetic fields, light-at-night, and nocturnal urinary 6-sulfatoxymelatonin concentration in women. *Am J Epidem.* 2001 Oct 1;154(7):591-600.

Davis S, Mirick DK, Stevens RG. Night shift work, light at night, and risk of breast cancer. *J Natl Cancer Inst.* 2001 Oct 17;93(20):1557-62.

Davis-Berman J, Berman DS. The widlerness therapy program: an empirical study of its effects with adolescents in an outpatient setting. *Journal of Contemporary Psychotherapy.* 1989;19 (4):271-281.

de Vries E, Coebergh JW, van der Rhee H. Trends, causes, approach and consequences related to the skin-cancer epidemic in the Netherlands and Europe. *Ned Tijdschr Geneeskd.* 2006 May 20;150(20):1108-15.

Dean E. Infrared measurements of healer-treated water. In: Roll W, Beloff J, White R (Eds.): *Research in parapsychology 1982.* Metuchen, NJ: Scarecrow Press, 1983:100-101.

Dement W, Vaughan C. *The Promise of Sleep.* New York: Dell, 1999.

Demers PA, Thomas DB, Rosenblatt KA, Jimenez LM, McTiernan A, Stalsberg H, Stemhagen A, Thompson WD, Curnen MG, Satariano W, *et al.* Occupational exposure to electromagnetic fields and breast cancer in men. *Am J Epidemiol.* 1991 Aug 15;134(4):340-7.

Deorah S, Lynch CF, Sibenaller ZA, Ryken TC. Trends in brain cancer incidence and survival in the US: Surveillance, Epidemiology, and End Results, 1973 to 2001. *Neurosrg Foc.* 2006 Apr 15;20(4):E1.

Diamond WJ, Cowden WL, Goldberg B. *Cancer Diagnosis: What to Do Next.* Tiburon, CA: AlternMed, 2000.

Dimbylow PJ, Mann SM. SAR calculations in an anatomically realistic model of the head for mobile communication transceivers at 900 MHz and 1.8 GHz. *Phys Med Biol.* 1994 Oct;39(10):1537-53.

Dimitriadis GD, Raptis SA. Thyroid hormone excess and glucose intolerance. *Exp Clin Endocrinol Diabetes.* 2001;109 Suppl 2:S225-39.

Dudley M. *Microwaved water and plants.* 2006; http://www.execonn.com/sf/. Accessed: 2007 Dec.

Ebbesen F, Agati G, Pratesi R. Phototherapy with turquoise versus blue light. *Arch Dis Child Fetal Neonatal Ed.* 2003 Sep;88(5):F430-1.

Edwards R, Ibison M, Jessel-Kenyon J, Taylor R. Light emission from the human body. *Comple Med Res.* 1989;3(2):16-19.

Edwards R, Ibison M, Jessel-Kenyon J, Taylor R. Measurements of human bioluminescence. *Acup Elect Res, Intl Jnl.* 1990;15:85-94.

Egan KM, Sosman JA, Blot WJ. Sunlight and reduced risk of cancer: is the real story vitamin D? *J Natl Cancer Inst.* 2005 Feb 2;97(3):161-3.

Einstein In Need Of Update? Calculations Show The Speed Of Light Might Change. *Science Daily.* 2001 Feb 12. www.sciencedaily.com/releases/ 2001/02/010212075309.htm. Accessed: 2007 Oct.

Electromagnetic fields: the biological evidence. *Science.* 1990;249:1378-1381.

Electronic Evidence of Auras, Chakras in UCLA Study. *Brain/Mind Bulletin.* 1978;3:9 Mar 20.

Eltiti S, Wallace D, Ridgewell A, Zougkou K, Russo R, Sepulveda F, *et al.* Does Short-Term Exposure to Mobile Phone Base Station Signals Increase Symptoms in Individuals who Report Sensitivity to Electromagnetic Fields? *Environ Health Perspect.* 2007;115(11):1603-1608.

Environmental Working Group. *Human Toxome Project.* 2007. http://www.ewg.org/sites/humantoxome/. Accessed: 2007 Sep.

EPA. *A Brief Guide to Mold, Moisture and Your Home.* Environmental Protection Agency, Office of Air and Radiation/Indoor Environments Division. EPA 2002;402-K-02-003.

Evans P, Forte D, Jacobs C, Fredhoi C, Aitchison E, Hucklebridge F, Clow A. Cortisol secretory activity in older people in relation to positive and negative well-being. *Psychoneuroendocrinology.* 2007 Aug 7.

Fan X, Zhang D, Zheng J, Gu N, Ding A, Jia X, Qing H, Jin L, Wan M, Li Q. Preparation and characterization of magnetic nano-particles with radiofrequency-induced hyperthermia for cancer treatment. *Sheng Wu Yi Xue Gong Cheng Xue Za Zhi.* 2006 Aug;23(4):809-13.

Fecher LA, Cummings SD, Keefe MJ, Alani RM. Toward a molecular classification of melanoma. *J Clin Oncol.* 2007 Apr 20;25(12):1606-20.

Fehring RJ, Schneider M, Raviele K. Variability in the phases of the menstrual cycle. *J Obstet Gynecol Neonatal Nurs.* 2006 May-Jun;35(3):376-84.

Felton JS, Fultz E, Dolbeare FA, Knize MG. Effect of microwave pretreatment on heterocyclic aromatic amine mutagens/carcinogens in fried beef patties. *Food Chem Toxicol.* 1994 Oct;32(10):897-903.

Fews AP, Henshaw DL, Keitch PA, Close JJ, Wilding RJ. Increased exposure to pollutant aerosols under high voltage power lines. *Int J Radiat Biol.* 1999 Dec;75(12):1505-21.

Field RW, Krewski D, Lubin JH, Zielinski JM, Alavanja M, Catalan VS, Klotz JB, Letourneau EG, Lynch CF, Lyon JL, Sandler DP, Schoenberg JB, Steck DJ, Stolwijk JA, Weinberg C, Wilcox HB. An overview of the North American residential radon and lung cancer case-control studies. *J Toxicol Environ Health A.* 2006 Apr;69(7):599-631.

Foer J, Siffre M. Caveman: An Interview with Michel Siffre. *Cabinet.* 2008 Summer (30).

Freeman HL, Stansfield SA. Psychosocial effects of urban environments, noise, and crowding. In Lundberg, A. (ed) *Environment and Mental Health.* London: Lawrence Erlbaum. 1998:147-173.

Frey A. Electromagnetic field interactions with biological systems. *FASEB Jnl.* 1993;7:272-28.

Fukada Y, Okano T. Circadian clock system in the pineal gland. *Mol Neurobiol.* 2002 Feb;25(1):19-30.

Galaev, YM. The Measuring of Ether-Drift Velocity and Kinematic Ether Viscosity within Optical Wave Bands. *Spacetime & Substance.* 2002;3(5):207-224.

Gambini JP, Velluti RA, Pedemonte M. Hippocampal theta rhythm synchronizes visual neurons in sleep and waking. *Brain Res.* 2002 Feb 1;926(1-2):137-41.

Gange R. UVA sunbeds - are there longterm hazards. In Cronley-Dillon J, Rosen E, Marshall J (Eds.):*Hazards of Light, Myths and Realities.* Oxford, U.K.: Pergamon Press, 1986.

García AM, Sisternas A, Hoyos SP. Occupational exposure to extremely low frequency electric and magnetic fields and Alzheimer disease: a meta-analysis. *Int J Epidemiol.* 2008 Apr;37(2):329-40.

Garcia-Lazaro JA, Ahmed B, Schnupp JW. Tuning to natural stimulus dynamics in primary auditory cortex. *Curr Biol.* 2006 Feb 7;16(3):264-71.

Garland CF, Gorham ED, Mohr SB, Grant WB, Giovannucci EL, Lipkin M, Newmark H, Holick MF, Garland FC. Vitamin D and prevention of breast cancer: pooled analysis. *J Steroid Biochem Mol Biol.* 2007 Mar;103(3-5):708-11.

Gau SS, Soong WT, Merikangas KR. Correlates of sleep-wake patterns among children and young adolescents in Taiwan. *Sleep.* 2004 May 1;27(3):512-9.

Gesler WM. Therapeutic landscapes: medical issues in light of the new cultural geography. *Soc Sci Med.* 1992 Apr;34(7):735-46.

Ghadioungui P. (transl.) *The Ebers Papyrus.* Academy of Scientific Research. Cairo, 1987.

Giovannucci E. The epidemiology of vitamin D and cancer incidence and mortality: *Cancer Causes Control.* 2005 Mar;16(2):83-95.

Goldstein LS, Dewhirst MW, Repacholi M, Kheifets L. Summary, conclusions and recommendations: adverse temperature levels in the human body. *Int J Hyperthermia.* 2003 May-Jun;19(3):373-84.

Goldstein N, Arshavskaya TV. Is atmospheric superoxide vitally necessary? Accelerated death of animals in a quasi-neutral electric atmosphere. *Z Naturforsch.* 1997. May-Jun;52(5-6):396-404.

Gomes A, Fernandes E, Lima JL. Fluorescence probes used for detection of reactive oxygen species. *J Biochem Biophys Methods.* 2005 Dec 31;65(2-3):45-80.

Gomez-Abellan P, Hernandez-Morante JJ, Lujan JA, Madrid JA, Garaulet M. Clock genes are implicated in the human metabolic syndrome. *Int J Obes.* 2007 Jul 24.

Gorham ED, Mohr SB, Garland CF, Chaplin G, Garland FC. Do sunscreens increase risk of melanoma in populations residing at higher latitudes? *Ann Epidemiol.* 2007 Dec;17(12):956-63.

Grad B, Dean E. Independent confirmation of infrared healer effects. In: White R, Broughton R (Eds.): *Research in parapsychology 1983.* Metuchen, NJ: Scarecrow Press, 1984:81-83.

Grad B. The 'Laying on of Hands': Implications for Psychotherapy, Gentling, and the Placebo Effect. *Jnl Amer Soc for Psych Res.* 1967 Oct;61(4):286-305.

Graham C, Sastre A, Cook MR, Kavet R, Gerkovich MM, Riffle DW. Exposure to strong ELF magnetic fields does not alter cardiac autonomic control mechanisms. *Bioelectromagnetics.* 2000 Sep;21(6):413-21.

Grant WB, Garland CF. The association of solar ultraviolet B (UVB) with reducing risk of cancer: multifactorial ecologic analysis of geographic variation in age-adjusted cancer mortality rates. *Anticancer Res.* 2006 Jul-Aug;26(4A):2687-99.

Grant WB, Holick MF. Benefits and requirements of vitamin D for optimal health: a review. *Altern Med Rev.* 2005 Jun;10(2):94-111.

Grant WB. An estimate of premature cancer mortality in the U.S. due to inadequate doses of solar ultraviolet-B radiation. *Cancer.* 2002 Mar 15;94(6):1867-75.

Grant WB. Solar ultraviolet irradiance and cancer incidence and mortality. *Adv Exp Med Biol.* 2008;624:16-30.

Grissom C. Magnetic field effects in biology: A survey of possible mechanisms with emphasis on radical pair recombination. *Chem. Rev.* 1995;95:3-24.

Gronfier C, Wright KP Jr, Kronauer RE, Czeisler CA. Entrainment of the human circadian pacemaker to longer-than-24-h days. *Proc Natl Acad Sci U S A.* 2007 May 22;104(21):9081-6.

Guerin M, Huntley ME, Olaizola M. Haematococcus astaxanthin: applications for human health and nutrition. *Trends Biotechnol.* 2003 May;21(5):210-6.

Gupta YK, Gupta M, Kohli K. Neuroprotective role of melatonin in oxidative stress vulnerable brain. *Indian J Physiol Pharmacol.* 2003 Oct;47(4):373-86.

Haarala C, Bergman M, Laine M, Revonsuo A, Koivisto M, Hamalainen H. Electromagnetic field emitted by 902 MHz mobile phones shows no effects on children's cognitive function. *Bioelectromagnetics.* 2005;Suppl 7:S144-50.

Hagins WA, Penn RD, Yoshikami S. Dark current and photocurrent in retinal rods. *Biophys J.* 1970 May;10(5):380-412.

Hagins WA, Robinson WE, Yoshikami S. Ionic aspects of excitation in rod outer segments. *Ciba Found Symp.* 1975;(31):169-89.

Hagins WA, Yoshikami S. Ionic mechanisms in excitation of photoreceptors. *Ann N Y Acad Sci.* 1975 Dec 30;264:314-25.

Hagins WA, Yoshikami S. Proceedings: A role for Ca2+ in excitation of retinal rods and cones. *Exp Eye Res.* 1974 Mar;18(3):299-305.

Hagins WA. The visual process: Excitatory mechanisms in the primary receptor cells. *Annu Rev Biophys Bioeng.* 1972;1:131-58.

Halliday GM, Agar NS, Barnetson RS, Ananthaswamy HN, Jones AM. UV-A fingerprint mutations in human skin cancer. *Photochem Photobiol.* 2005 Jan-Feb;81(1):3-8.

Halpern S. *Tuning the Human Instrument.* Palo Alto, CA: Spectrum Research Institute, 1978.

Hammermeister J, Brock B, Winterstein D, Page R. Life without TV? cultivation theory and psychosocial health characteristics of television-free individuals and their television-viewing counterparts. *Health Commun.* 2005;17(3):253-64.

Hammitt WE. The relation between being away and privacy in urban forest recreation environments. *Environment and Behaviour.* 2000;32 (4):521-540.

Hancox RJ, Milne BJ, Poulton R. Association of television viewing during childhood with poor educational achievement. *Arch Pediatr Adolesc Med.* 2005 Jul;159(7):614-8.

Handwerk B. Are Earthquakes Encouraged by High Tides? *National Geographic News.* 2004 Oct 22.

Hanifin JP, Stewart KT, Smith P, Tanner R, Rollag M, Brainard GC. High-intensity red light suppresses melatonin. *Chronobiol Int.* 2006;23(1-2):251-68.

Hans J. *The Structure and Dynamics of Waves and Vibrations.* New York:.Schocken and Co., 1975.

Hardin P. Transcription regulation within the circadian clock: the E-box and beyond. *J Biol Rhythms.* 2004 Oct;19(5):348-60.

Harkins T, Grissom C. Magnetic Field Effects on B12 Ethanolamine Ammonia Lyase: Evidence for a Radical Mechanism. *Science.* 1994;263:958-960.

Harkins T, Grissom C. The Magnetic Field Dependent Step in B12 Ethanolamine Ammonia Lyase is Radical-Pair Recombination. *J. Am. Chem. Soc.* 1995;117:566-567.

Harland JD, Liburdy RP. Environmental magnetic fields inhibit the antiproliferative action of tamoxifen and melatonin in a human breast cancer cell line. *Bioelectromagnetics.* 1997;18(8):555-62.

Harris RB, Foote JA, Hakim IA, Bronson DL, Alberts DS. Fatty acid composition of red blood cell membranes and risk of squamous cell carcinoma of the skin. *Cancer Epidemiol Biomarkers Prev.* 2005 Apr;14(4):906-12.

Heaney RP, Recker RR, Grote J, Horst RL, Armas LA. Vitamin D(3) is more potent than vitamin D(2) in humans. J Clin Endocrinol Metab. 2011 Mar;96(3):E447-52. doi: 10.1210/jc.2010-2230.

Heerwagen JH. The psychological aspects of windows and window design'. In Selby, R. I., Anthony, K. H., Choi, J. and Orland, B. (eds) *Proceedings of 21st Annual Conference of the Environmental Design Research Association.* Champaign-Urbana, Illinois, 1990 April:6-9.

Heinrich U, Gärtner C, Wiebusch M, Eichler O, Sies H, Tronnier H, Stahl W. Supplementation with beta-carotene or a similar amount of mixed carotenoids protects humans from UV-induced erythema. *J Nutr.* 2003 Jan;133(1):98-101.

Henderson SI, Bangay MJ. Survey of RF exposure levels from mobile telephone base stations in Australia. *Bioelectromag.* 2006 Jan;27(1):73-6.

Henshaw DL, Ross AN, Fews AP, Preece AW. Enhanced deposition of radon daughter nuclei in the vicinity of power frequency electromagnetic fields. *Int J Radiat Biol.* 1996 Jan;69(1):25-38.

Hess AF. *Rickets.* London: Henry Kimpton, 1930.

Heyers D, Manns M, Luksch H, Gü"ntü" rku"n O, Mouritsen H. A Visual Pathway Links Brain Structures Active during Magnetic Compass Orientation in Migratory Birds. *PLoS One.* 2007;2(9):e937. 2007.

Hietanen M, Hamalainen AM, Husman T. Hypersensitivity symptoms associated with exposure to cellular telephones: no causal link. *Bioelectromagnetics.* 2002 May;23(4):264-70.

Hirayama J, Sahar S, Grimaldi B, Tamaru T, Takamatsu K, Nakahata Y, Sassone-Corsi P. CLOCK-mediated acetylation of BMAL1 controls circadian function. *Nature* 450, 1086-1090 (13 December 2007)

Hjollund NH, Bonde JP, Skotte J. Semen analysis of personnel operating military radar equipment. *Reprod Toxicol.* 1997 Nov-Dec;11(6):897.

Holick MF. Photobiology of vitamin D. In: Feldman D, Pike JW, Glorieux FH, eds. *Vitamin D,* Second Edition, Volume I. Burlington, MA: Elsevier, 2005.

Holick MF. Sunlight and vitamin D for bone health and prevention of autoimmune diseases, cancers, and cardiovascular disease. *Am J Clin Nutr.* 2004 Dec;80(6 Suppl):1678S-88S.

Holick MF. Vitamin D status: measurement, interpretation, and clinical application. Ann Epidemiol. 2009 Feb;19(2):73-8.

Holick MF. Vitamin D. In: Shils ME, Shike M, Ross AC, Caballero B, Cousins RJ, eds. *Modern Nutrition in Health and Disease,* 10th ed. Philadelphia: Lippincott Williams & Wilkins, 2006.

Holick MF. Vitamin D: importance in the prevention of cancers, type 1 diabetes, heart disease, and osteoporosis. *Am J Clin Nutr.* 2004 Mar;79(3):362-71.

Hollfoth K. Effect of color therapy on health and wellbeing: colors are more than just physics. *Pflege.Z* 2000;53(2):111-112.

Hollwich F, Dieckhues B, Schrameyer B. The effect of natural and artificial light via the eye on the hormonal and metabolic balance of man. *Klin Monbl Augenheilkd.* 1977 Jul;171(1):98-104.

Hollwich F, Dieckhues B. Effect of light on the eye on metabolism and hormones. *Klin Monbl Augenheilkd.* 1989 Nov;195(5):284-90.

Hollwich F, Hartmann C. Influence of light through the eyes on metabolism and hormones. *Ophtalmologie.* 1990 Jul-Aug;4(4):385-9.

Hollwich F. *The influence of ocular light perception on metabolism in man and in animal.* NY: Springer-Verlag, 1979.

Holly EA, Aston DA, Ahn DK, Smith AH. Intraocular melanoma linked to occupations and chemical exposures. *Epidemiology.* 1996 Jan;7(1):55-61.

Holman CD, Armstrong BK, Heenan PJ. Relationship of cutaneous malignant melanoma to individual sunlight-exposure habits. *J Natl Cancer Inst.* 1986 Mar;76(3):403-14.

Honeyman MK. Vegetation and stress: a comparison study of varying amounts of vegetation in countryside and urban scenes. In Relf, D. (ed) *The Role of Horticulture in Human Well-Being and Social Development: A National Symposium.* Portland: Timber Press. 1992:143-145.

Hood W, Nicholas J, Butler G, Lackland D, Hoel D, Mohr L. Magnetic field exposure of commercial airline pilots. *Annals of Epidemiology* 2000 Oct 1;10(7):479.

Horne JA, Donlon J, Arendt J. Green light attenuates melatonin output and sleepiness during sleep deprivation. *Sleep.* 1991 Jun;14(3):233-40.

Hoskin M.(ed.). *The Cambridge Illustrated History of Astronomy.* Cambridge: Cambridge Press, 1997.

Huesmann LR, Moise-Titus J, Podolski CL, Eron LD. Longitudinal relations between children's exposure to TV violence and their aggressive and violent behavior in young adulthood: 1977-1992. *Dev Psychol.* 2003 Mar;39(2):201-21.

Huffman C. Archytas of Tarentum: *Pythagorean, philosopher and Mathematician King.* Cambridge: Cambridge University Press, 2005.

Igarashi T, Izumi H, Uchiumi T, Nishio K, Arao T, Tanabe M, Uramoto H, Sugio K, Yasumoto K, Sasaguri Y, Wang KY, Otsuji Y, Kohno K. Clock and ATF4 transcription system regulates drug resistance in human cancer cell lines. *Oncogene.* 2007 Jul 19;26(33):4749-60.

Ikeda M, Toyoshima R, Inoue Y, Yamada N, Mishima K, Nomura M, Ozaki N, Okawa M, Takahashi K, Yamauchi T. Mutation screening of the human Clock gene in circadian rhythm sleep disorders. *Psychiatry Res.* 2002 Mar 15;109(2):121-8.

Ikonomov OC, Stoynev AG. Gene expression in suprachiasmatic nucleus and circadian rhythms. *Neurosci Biobehav Rev.* 1994 Fall;18(3):305-12.

Inaba H. INABA Biophoton. Exploratory Research for Advanced Technology. *Japan Science and Technology Agency.* 1991. http://www.jst.go.jp/erato/project/isf_P/isf_P.html. Accessed: 2006 Nov.

Ivry GB, Ogle CA, Shim EK. Role of sun exposure in melanoma. *Dermatol Surg.* 2006 Apr;32(4):481-92.

Jagetia GC, Aggarwal BB. "Spicing up" of the immune system by curcumin. *J Clin Immunol.* 2007 Jan;27(1):19-35.

Janssen S, Solomon G, Schettler T. Chemical Contaminants and Human Disease: *The Collaborative on Health and the Environment.* 2006. http://www.healthandenvironment.org. Accessed: 2007 Jul.

Jenab M, Bueno-de-Mesquita HB, Ferrari P, van Duijnhoven FJ, Norat T, Pischon T, Jansen EH, Slimani N, Byrnes G, Rinaldi S, Tjønneland A, Olsen A, Overvad K, Boutron-Ruault MC, Clavel-Chapelon F, Morois S, Kaaks R, Linseisen J, Boeing H, Bergmann MM, Trichopoulou A, Misirli G, Trichopoulos D, Berrino F, Vineis P, Panico S, Palli D, Tumino R, Ros MM, van Gils CH, Peeters PH, Brustad M, Lund E, Tormo MJ, Ardanaz E, Rodríguez L, Sánchez MJ, Dorronsoro M, Gonzalez CA, Hallmans G, Palmqvist R, Roddam A, Key TJ, Khaw KT, Autier P, Hainaut P, Riboli E. Association between pre-diagnostic circulating vitamin D concentration and risk of colorectal cancer in European populations: a nested case-control study. BMJ. 2010 Jan 21;340:b5500. doi: 10.1136/bmj.b5500.

Jensen B. *Foods that Heal.* Garden City Park, NY: Avery Publ, 1988, 1993.

Jensen B. *Nature Has a Remedy.* Los Angeles: Keats, 2001.

Johansen C. Electromagnetic fields and health effects – epidemiologic studies of cancer, diseases of the central nervous system and arrhythmia-related heart disease. *Scand J Work Env Hlth.* 2004;30 Spl 1:1-30.

Johansen C. Rehabilitation of cancer patients - research perspectives. *Acta Oncol.* 2007;46(4):441-5.

Johari H. *Ayurvedic Massage: Traditional Indian Techniques for Balancing Body and Mind.* Roch: Healing Arts, 1996.

Johari H. *Chakras.* Rochester, VT: Destiny, 1987.

Jovanovic-Ignjatic Z, Rakovic D. A review of current research in microwave resonance therapy: novel opportunities in medical treatment. *Acupunct Electrother Res.* 1999; 24:105-125.

Jovanovic-Ignjatic Z. Microwave Resonant Therapy: Novel Opportunities in Medical Treatment. *Acup. & Electro-Therap. Res., The Int. J.* 1999;24(2):105-125.

Jurkovicová I, Celec P. Sleep apnea syndrome and its complications. *Acta Med Austr.* 2004 May;31(2):45-50.

Kalsbeek A, Perreau-Lenz S, Buijs RM. A network of (autonomic) clock outputs. *Chronobiol Int.* 2006;23(1-2):201-15.

Kamide Y. We reside in the sun's atmosphere. *Biomed Pharmacother.* 2005 Oct;59 Suppl 1:S1-4.

Kamycheva E, Jorde R, Figenschau Y, Haug E. Insulin sensitivity in subjects with secondary hyperparathyroidism and the effect of a low serum 25-hydroxyvitamin D level on insulin sensitivity. J *Endocrinol Invest.* 2007 Feb;30(2):126-32.

Kandel E, Siegelbaum S, Schwartz J. *Synaptic transmission. Principles of Neural Science.* New York: Elsevier, 1991.

Kaplan R. The psychological benefits of nearby nature. In: Relf, D. (ed) *The Role of Horticulture in Human Well-Being and Social Development: A National Symposium.* Portland: Timber Press. 1992:125-133.

Kaplan S. A model of person - environment compatibility. *Environment and Behaviour* 1983;15:311-332.

Kaplan S. The restorative environment: nature and human experience. In: Relf, D. (ed) *The Role of Horticulture in Human Well-Being and Social Development: A National Symposium.* Portland: Timber Press. 1992:134-142.

Karis TE, Jhon MS. Flow-induced anisotropy in the susceptibility of a particle suspension. *Proc Natl Acad Sci USA.* 1986 Jul;83(14):4973-4977.

Karpin VA, Kostriukova NK, Gudkov AB. Human radiation action of radon and its daughter disintegration products. *Gig Sanit.* 2005 Jul-Aug;(4):13-7.

Kato Y, Kawamoto T, Honda KK. Circadian rhythms in cartilage. *Clin Calcium.* 2006 May;16(5):838-45.

Kelly TL, Neri DF, Grill JT, Ryman D, Hunt PD, Dijk DJ, Shanahan TL, Czeisler CA. Nonentrained circadian rhythms of melatonin in submariners scheduled to an 18-hour day. *J Biol Rhythms.* 1999 Jun;14(3):190-6.

Kent ST, McClure LA, Crosson WL, Arnett DK, Wadley VG, Sathiakumar N. Effect of sunlight exposure on cognitive function among depressed and non-depressed participants: a REGARDS cross-sectional study. *Environ Health.* 2009 Jul 28;8:34.

Khan S. Vitamin D deficiency and secondary hyperparathyroidism among patients with chronic kidney disease. *Am J Med Sci.* 2007 Apr;333(4):201-7.

Kheifets L, Monroe J, Vergara X, Mezei G, Afifi AA. Occupational electromagnetic fields and leukemia and brain cancer: an update to two meta-analyses. *J Occup Environ Med.* 2008 Jun;50(6):677-88.

Kinoshameg SA, Persinger MA. Suppression of experimental allergic encephalomyelitis in rats by 50-nT, 7-Hz amplitude-modulated nocturnal magnetic fields depends on when after inoculation the fields are applied. *Neurosci Lett.* 2004 Nov 11;370(2-3):166-70.

Kirlian SD, Kirlian V. Photography and Visual Observation by Means of High-Frequency Currents. *J Sci Appl Photogr.* 1963;6(6).

Kiyose C, *et al.* Biodiscrimination of alpha-tocopherol stereoisomers in humans after oral administration. *Am J Clin Nutr.* 1997 Mar; 65 (3):785-9.

Kleffmann J. Daytime Sources of Nitrous Acid (HONO) in the Atmospheric Boundary Layer. *Chemphyschem.* 2007 Apr 10;8(8):1137-1144.

Klein R, Armitage R. Rhythms in human performance: 1 1/2-hour oscillations in cognitive style. *Science.* 1979 Jun 22;204(4399):1326-8.

Kleitman N. *Sleep and Wakefulness.* Univ Chicago Press, 1963.

Kloss J. *Back to Eden.* Twin Oaks, WI: Lotus Press, 1939-1999.

Kniazeva TA, Kuznetsova LN, Otto MP, Nikiforova TI. Efficacy of chromotherapy in patients with hypertension. *Vopr Kurortol Fizioter Lech Fiz Kult.* 2006 Jan-Feb;(1):11-3.

Knize MG, Salmon CP, Pais P, Felton JS. Food heating and the formation of heterocyclic aromatic amine and polycyclic aromatic hydrocarbon mutagens/carcinogens. *Adv Exp Med Biol.* 1999;459:179-93.

Kollerstrom N, Staudenmaier G. Evidence for Lunar-Sidereal Rhythms in Crop Yield: A Review. *Biolog Agri & Hort.* 2001;19:247–259.

Köpcke W, Krutmann J. Protection from sunburn with beta-Carotene – a meta-analysis. *Photochem Photobiol.* 2008 Mar-Apr;84(2):284-8.

Kowalczyk E, Krzesiński P, Kura M, Niedworok J, Kowalski J, Błaszczyk J. Pharmacological effects of flavonoids from Scutellaria baicalensis. *Przegl Lek.* 2006;63(2):95-6.

Krause R, Buhring M, Hopfenmuller W, Holick MF, Sharma AM. Ultraviolet B and blood pressure. *Lancet.* 1998 Aug 29;352(9129):709-10.

Küller R, Laike T. The impact of flicker from fluorescent lighting on well-being, performance and physiological arousal. *Ergonomics.* 1998 Apr;41(4):433-47.

Kuribayashi M, Wang J, Fujiwara O, Doi Y, Nabae K, Tamano S, Ogiso T, Asamoto M, Shirai T. Lack of effects of 1439 MHz electromagnetic near field exposure on the blood-brain barrier in immature and young rats. *Bioelectromagnetics.* 2005 Oct;26(7):578-88.

Kuuler R, Ballal S, Laike T Mikellides B, Tonello G. The impact of light and colour on psychological mood: a cross-cultral study of indoor work environments. *Ergonomics.* 2006 Nov 15;49(14):1496.

Lad V. *Ayurveda: The Science of Self-Healing.* Twin Lakes, WI: Lotus Press.

Lafrenière, G. The material Universe is made purely out of Aether. *Matter is made of Waves.* 2002. http://www.glafreniere.com/matter.htm. Accessed: 2007 June.

Lakin-Thomas PL. Transcriptional feedback oscillators: maybe, maybe not. *J Bio Rhyth.* 2006 Apr;21(2):83-92.

Lancranjan I, Maicanescu M, Rafaila E, Klepsch I, Popescu HI. Gonadic function in workmen with long-term exposure to microwaves. *Health Phys.* 1975;29:381–383.

Lappe JM, Travers-Gustafson D, Davies KM, Recker RR, Heaney RP. Vitamin D and calcium supplementation reduces cancer risk: results of a randomized trial. *Am J Clin Nutr.* 2007 Jun;85(6):1586-91.

Larsen AI, Olsen J, Svane O. Gender-specific reproductive outcome and exposure to high-frequency electromagnetic radiation among physiotherapists. *Scand J Work Environ Health.* 1991;17:324–329.

Larsen AI, Skotte J. Can exposure to electromagnetic radiation in diathermy operators be estimated from interview data? A pilot study. *Am J Ind Med* 1991;19:51–57.

Larsen AI. Congenital malformations and exposure to high-frequency electromagnetic radiation among Danish physiotherapists. *Scand J Work Environ Health.* 1991;17:318–323.

Laverty WH, Kelly IW. Cyclical calendar and lunar patterns in automobile property accidents and injury accidents. *Percept Mot Skills.* 1998 Feb;86(1):299-302.

Lee KR, Kozukue N, Han JS, Park JH, Chang EY, Baek EJ, Chang JS, Friedman M. Glycoalkaloids and metabolites inhibit the growth of human colon (HT29) and liver (HepG2) cancer cells. *J Agric Food Chem.* 2004 May 19;52(10):2832-9.

Lehmann B. The vitamin D3 pathway in human skin and its role for regulation of biological processes. *Photochem Photobiol.* 2005 Nov-Dec;81(6):1246-51.

Lenn NJ, Beebe B, Moore RY (1977) Postnatal development of the suprachiasmatic nucleus of the rat. *Cell Tissue Res.* 178:463-475.

Leroux E, Ducros A. Cluster headache. *Orphanet J Rare Dis.* 2008 Jul 23;3:20.

Li DK, Odouli R, Wi S, Janevic T, Golditch I, Bracken TD, Senior R, Rankin R, Iriye R. A population-based prospective cohort study of personal exposure to magnetic fields during pregnancy and the risk of miscarriage. *Epidemiology.* 2002 Jan;13(1):9-20.

Li Q, Gandhi OP. Calculation of magnetic field-induced current densities for humans from EAS countertop activation/deactivation devices that use ferromagnetic cores. *Phys Med Biol.* 2005 Jan 21;50(2):373-85.

Lieber AL. Human aggression and the lunar synodic cycle. *J Clin Psychiatry.* 1978 May;39(5):385-92.

Livanova L, Levshina I, Nozdracheva L, Elbakidze MG, Airapetiants MG. The protective action of negative air ions in acute stress in rats with different typological behavioral characteristics. *Zh Vyssh Nerv Deiat Im I P Pavlova.* 1998 May-Jun;48(3):554-7.

Lloyd D, Murray D. Redox rhythmicity: clocks at the core of temporal coherence.*BioEss.* 2007;29(5):465-473.

Lloyd JU. *American Materia Medica, Therapeutics and Pharmacognosy.* Portland, OR: Eclect Med Publ, 1989-1983.

Loughnan ME, Nicholls N, Tapper NJ. Demographic, seasonal, and spatial differences in acute myocardial infarction admissions to hospital in Melbourne Australia. *Int J Health Geogr.* 2008 Jul 30;7:42.

Lovejoy S, Pecknold S, Schertzer D. Stratified multifractal magnetization and surface geomagnetic fields – I. Spectral analysis and modeling. *Geophysical Journal International.* 2001;145(1):112-126.

Loving RT, Kripke DF, Knickerbocker NC, Grandner MA. Bright green light treatment of depression for older adults. *BMC Psychiatry.* 2005 Nov 9;5:42.

Lydic R, Schoene WC, Czeisler CA, Moore-Ede MC. Suprachiasmatic region of the human hypothalamus: homolog to the primate circadian pacemaker? *Sleep.* 1980;2(3):355-61.

Lythgoe JN. Visual pigments and environmental light. *Vision Res.* 1984;24(11):1539-50.

Maas J, Jayson, J. K.. & Kleiber, D. A. Effects of spectral differences in illumination on fatigue. *J Appl Psychol.* 1974;59:524-526.

Maccabee PJ, Amassian VE, Cracco RQ, Cracco JB, Eberle L, Rudell A. Stimulation of the human nervous system using the magnetic coil. *J Clin Neurophysiol.* 1991 Jan;8(1):38-55.

Magnusson A, Stefansson JG. Prevalence of seasonal affective disorder in Iceland. *Arch Gen Psychiatry.* 1993 Dec;50(12):941-6.

Maier R, Greter SE, Maier N. Effects of pulsed electromagnetic fields on cognitive processes - a pilot study on pulsed field interference with cognitive regeneration. *Acta Neurol Scand.* 2004 Jul;110(1):46-52.

Maier T, Korting HC. Sunscreens - which and what for? *Skin Pharmacol Physiol.* 2005 Nov-Dec;18(6):253-62.

Makomaski Illing EM, Kaiserman MJ. Mortality attributable to tobacco use in Canada and its regions, 1998. *Can J Public Health.* 2004;95(1):38-44.

Mansour HA, Monk TH, Nimgaonkar VL. Circadian genes and bipolar disorder. *Ann Med.* 2005;37(3):196-205.

Marasanov SB, Matveev II. Correlation between protracted premedication and complication in cancer patients operated on during intense solar activity. *Vopr Onkol.* 2007;53(1):96-9.

Mastorakos G, Pavlatou M. Exercise as a stress model and the interplay between the hypothalamus-pituitary-adrenal and the hypothalamus-pituitary-thyroid axes. *Horm Metab Res.* 2005 Sep;37(9):577-84.

Matsumura Y, Nishigori C, Yagi T, Imamura S, Takebe H. Characterization of p53 gene mutations in basal-cell carcinomas: comparison between sun-exposed and less-exposed skin areas. *Int J Cancer.* 1996 Mar 15;65(6):778-80.

Matutinovic Z, Galic M. Relative magnetic hearing threshold. *Laryngol Rhinol Otol.* 1982 Jan;61(1):38-41.

Mayron L, Ott J, Nations R, Mayron E. Light, radiation and academic behaviour: Initial studies on the effects of full-spectrum lighting and radiation shielding on behaviour and academic performance of school children. *Acad Ther.* 1974;10, 33-47.

Mayron L. Hyperactivity from fluorescent lighting - fact or fancy: A commentary on the report by O'Leary, Rosenbaum and Hughes. *J Abnorm Child Psychol.* 1978;6:291-294.

McClung CA. Role for the Clock gene in bipolar disorder. *Cold Spring Harb Symp Quant Biol.* 2007;72:637-44.

McColl SL, Veitch JA. Full-spectrum fluorescent lighting: a review of its effects on physiology and health. *Psychol Med.* 2001 Aug;31(6):949-64.

McLay RN, Daylo AA, Hammer PS. No effect of lunar cycle on psychiatric admissions or emergency evaluations. *Mil Med.* 2006 Dec;171(12):1239-42.

Mendoza J. Circadian clocks: setting time by food. *J Neuroendocrinol.* 2007 Feb;19(2):127-37.

Merchant RE and Andre CA. 2001. A review of recent clinical trials of the nutritional supplement Chlorella pyrenoidosa in the treatment of fibromyalgia, hypertension, and ulcerative colitis. *Altern Ther Health Med.* May-Jun;7(3):79-91.

Miles LE, Raynal DM, Wilson MA. Blind man living in normal society has circadian rhythms of 24.9 hours. *Science.* 1977 Oct 28;198(4315):421-3.

Millen AE, Tucker MA, Hartge P, Halpern A, Elder DE, Guerry D 4th, Holly EA, Sagebiel RW, Potischman N. Diet and melanoma in a case-control study. *Cancer Epidem Biomarkers Prev.* 2004 Jun;13(6):1042-51.

Miller GT. *Living in the Environment.* Belmont, CA: Wadsworth, 1996.

Miller JD, Morin LP, Schwartz WJ, Moore RY. New insights into the mammalian circadian clock. *Sleep.* 1996 Oct;19(8):641-67.

Mohr SB, Garland CF, Gorham ED, Grant WB, Garland FC. Is ultraviolet B irradiance inversely associated with incidence rates of endometrial cancer: an ecological study of 107 countries. *Prev Med.* 2007 Nov;45(5):327-31.

Mohr SB. A brief history of vitamin d and cancer prevention. *Ann Epidemiol.* 2009 Feb;19(2):79-83.

Moore R. Circadian Rhythms: A Clock for the Ages. Science 1999 June 25;284(5423):2102 – 2103.

Moore RY, Speh JC. Serotonin innervation of the primate suprachiasmatic nucleus. *Brain Res.* 2004 Jun 4;1010(1-2):169-73.

Moore RY. Neural control of the pineal gland. *Behav Brain Res.* 1996;73(1-2):125-30.

Moore RY. Organization and function of a central nervous system circadian oscillator: the suprachiasmatic hypothalamic nucleus. *Fed Proc.* 1983 Aug;42(11):2783-9.

Moorhead KJ, Morgan HC. *Spirulina: Nature's Superfood.* Kailua-Kona, HI: Nutrex, 1995.

Morton C. *Velocity Alters Electric Field.* www.amasci.com/ freenrg/ morton1.html. Accessed: 2007 July.

Murchie G. *The Seven Mysteries of Life.* Boston: Houghton Mifflin Company, 1978.

Musaev AV, Nasrullaeva SN, Zeïnalov RG. Effects of solar activity on some demographic indices and morbidity in Azerbaijan with reference to A. L. Chizhevsky's theory. *Vopr Kurortol Fizioter Lech Fiz Kult.* 2007 May-Jun;(3):38-42.

Nadkarni AK, Nadkarni KM. *Indian Materia Medica.* (Vols 1 and 2). Bombay: Popular Pradashan, 1908, 1976.

Nakatani K, Yau KW. Calcium and light adaptation in retinal rods and cones. *Nature.* 1988 Jul 7;334(6177): 69-71.

Napoli N, Thompson J, Civitelli R, Villareal R. Effects of dietary calcium compared with calcium supplements on estrogen metabolism and bone mineral density. *Am J Clin Nutr.* 2007;85(5): 1428-1433.

Natarajan E, Grissom C. The Origin of Magnetic Field Dependent Recombination in Alkylcobalamin Radical Pairs. *Photochem Photobiol.* 1996;64: 286-295.

Navarro Silvera SA, Rohan TE. Trace elements and cancer risk: a review of the epidemiologic evidence. *Cancer Causes Control.* 2007 Feb;18(1):7-27.

Nicholas JS, Lackland DT, Butler GC, Mohr LC Jr, Dunbar JB, Kaune WT, Grosche B, Hoel DG. Cosmic radiation and magnetic field exposure to airline flight crews. *Am J Ind Med.* 1998 Dec;34(6):574-80.

Nielsen LR, Mosekilde L. Vitamin D and breast cancer. *Ugeskr Laeger.* 2007 Apr 2;169(14):1299-302.

Nievergelt CM, Kripke DF, Remick RA, Sadovnick AD, McElroy SL, Keck PE Jr, Kelsoe JR. Examination of the clock gene Cryptochrome 1 in bipolar disorder: mutational analysis and absence of evidence for linkage or association. *Psychiatr Genet.* 2005 Mar;15(1):45-52.

Nishigori C, Hattori Y, Toyokuni S. Role of reactive oxygen species in skin carcinogenesis. *Antioxid Redox Signal.* 2004 Jun;6(3):561-70.

North J. *The Fontana History of Astronomy and Cosmology.* London: Fontana Press, 1994.

NRPB 2003. Health Effects from Radiofrequency Electromagnetic Fields. Report of an Independent Advisory Group on Non-ionising Radiation. Chilton, Didcot, *UK:National Radiation Protection Board.*

Núñez S, Pérez Méndez L, Aguirre-Jaime A. Moon cycles and violent behaviours: myth or fact? *Eur J Emerg Med.* 2002 Jun;9(2):127-30.

Okamura H. Clock genes in cell clocks: roles, actions, and mysteries. *J Biol Rhythms.* 2004 Oct;19(5):388-99.

Ole D. Rughede, On the Theory and Physics of the Aether. *Progress in Physics.* 2006; (1).

O'Leary KD, Rosenbaum A, Hughes PC. Fluorescent lighting: a purported source of hyperactive behavior. *J Abnorm Child Psychol.* 1978 Sep;6(3):285-9.

Otsu A, Chinami M, Morgenthale S, Kaneko Y, Fujita D, Shirakawa T. Correlations for number of sunspots, unemployment rate, and suicide mortality in Japan. Percept Mot Skills. 2006 Apr;102(2):603-8.

Ouellet-Hellstrom R, Stewart WF. Miscarriages among female physical therapists who report using radio- and microwave-frequency electromagnetic radiation. *Am J Epidemiol.* 1993 Nov 15;138(10):775-86.

Owen C, Tarantello C, Jones M, Tennant C. Lunar cycles and violent behaviour. *Aust-NZ J Psych.*1998 Aug;32(4):496-9.

Ozone Hole Healing Gradually. *Associated Press.* 2005 Sept 16, 03:18 pm ET.

Paavonen EJ, Pennonen M, Roine M, Valkonen S, Lahikainen AR. TV exposure associated with sleep disturbances in 5- to 6-year-old children. J Sleep Res. 2006 Jun;15(2):154-61.

Pacione M. Urban environmental quality and human wellbeing-a social geographical perspective. *Landscape and Urban Planning* 2003;986:1-12.

Palm TA. The geographical distribution and aetiology of rickets. *Practitioner.* 1890;45:270-90, 321-42.

Palumbo A. Gravitational and geomagnetic tidal source of earthquake triggering. *Ital Phys.* 1989 Nov;12(6).

Partonen T, Haukka J, Nevanlinna H, Lönnqvist J. Analysis of the seasonal pattern in suicide. *J Affect Disord.* 2004 Aug;81(2):133-9.

Partonen T, Haukka J, Viilo K, Hakko H, Pirkola S, Isometsä E, Lönnqvist J, Särkioja T, Väisänen E, Räsänen P. Cyclic time patterns of death from suicide in N. Finland. *J Affect Disrd.* 2004 Jan;78(1):11-9.

Partonen T. Magnetoreception attributed to the efficacy of light therapy. *Med Hypoth.* 1998 Nov;51(5):447-8.

Pedemonte M, Rodríguez-Alvez A, Velluti RA. Electroencephalographic frequencies associated with heart changes in RR interval variability during paradoxical sleep. *Auton Neurosci.* 2005 Dec 30;123(1-2):82-6.

Penev PD. Association between sleep and morning testosterone levels in older men. *Sleep.* 2007 Apr 1;30(4):427-32.

Penn RD, Hagins WA. Kinetics of the photocurrent of retinal rods. *Biophys J.* 1972 Aug;12(8):1073-94.

Penn RD, Hagins WA. Signal transmission along retinal rods and the origin of the electroretinographic a-wave. *Nature.* 1969 Jul 12;223(5202):201-4.

Pérez-López FR. Vitamin D and its implications for musculoskeletal health in women: an update. *Maturitas.* 2007 Oct 20;58(2):117-37.

Peroxisomes from pepper fruits (Capsicum annuum L.): purification, characterisation and antioxidant activity. *J Plant Physiol.* 2003 Dec;160(12):1507-16.

Perreau-Lenz S, Kalsbeek A, Van Der Vliet J, Pevet P, Buijs RM. In vivo evidence for a controlled offset of melatonin synthesis at dawn by the suprachiasmatic nucleus in the rat. *Neurosci.* 2005;130(3):797-803.

Perrin RN. Lymphatic drainage of the neuraxis in chronic fatigue syndrome: a hypothetical model for the cranial rhythmic impulse. *J Am Osteopath Assoc.* 2007 Jun;107(6):218-24.

Persson R, Orbaek P, Kecklund G, Akerstedt T. Impact of an 84-hour workweek on biomarkers for stress, metabolic processes and diurnal rhythm. *Scand J Work Environ Health.* 2006 Oct;32(5):349-58.

Piggins HD. Human clock genes. *Ann Med.* 2002;34(5):394-400.

Piluso LG, Moffatt-Smith C. Disinfection using ultraviolet radiation as an antimicrobial agent: a review and synthesis of mechanisms and concerns. PDA J Pharm Sci Technol. 2006 Jan-Feb;60(1):1-16.

Pittas AG, Harris SS, Stark PC, Dawson-Hughes B. The effects of calcium and vitamin D supplementation on blood glucose and markers of inflammation in nondiabetic adults. *Diab Care.* 2007 Apr;30(4):980-6.

Pitt-Rivers R, Trotter WR. *The Thyroid Gland.* London: Butterworth Publisher, 1954.

Plotnikoff GA, Quigley JM. Prevalence of severe hypovitaminosis D in patients with persistent, nonspecific musculoskeletal pain. Mayo Clin Proc 2003;78: 1463-70.

Ponsonby AL, McMichael A, van der Mei I. Ultraviolet radiation and autoimmune disease: insights from epidemiological research. *Toxicology.* 2002 Dec 27;181-182:71-8.

Pont AR, Charron AR, Brand RM. Active ingredients in sunscreens act as topical penetration enhancers for the herbicide 2,4-dichlorophenoxyacetic acid. *Toxicol Appl Pharmacol.* 2004 Mar 15;195(3):348-54.

Pool R. Is there an EMF-Cancer connection? *Science.* 1990;249: 1096-1098.

Portaluppi F, Hermida RC. Circadian rhythms in cardiac arrhythmias and opportunities for their chronotherapy. *Adv Drug Deliv Rev.* 2007 Aug 31;59(9-10):940-51.

Prato FS, Frappier JR, Shivers RR, Kavaliers M, Zabel P, Drost D, Lee TY. Magnetic resonance imaging increases the blood-brain barrier permeability to 153-gadolinium diethylenetriaminepentaacetic acid in rats. *Brain Res.* 1990 Jul 23;523(2):301-4.

Preisinger E, Quittan M. Thermo- and hydrotherapy. *Wien Med Wochenschr.* 1994;144(20-21):520-6.

Pronina TS. Circadian and infradian rhythms of testosterone and aldosterone excretion in children. *Probl Endokrinol.* 1992 Sep-Oct;38(5):38-42.

Ravindra T, Lakshmi NK, Ahuja YR. Melatonin in pathogenesis and therapy of cancer. *Indian J Med Sci.* 2006 Dec;60(12):523-35.

Regel SJ, Negovetic S, Roosli M, Berdinas V, Schuderer J, Huss A, *et al.* UMTS base station-like exposure, well-being, and cognitive performance. *Environ Health Perspect.* 2006 Aug;114(8):1270-5.

Reichrath J. The challenge resulting from positive and negative effects of sunlight: how much solar UV exposure is appropriate to balance between risks of vitamin D deficiency and skin cancer? *Prog Biophys Mol Biol.* 2006 Sep;92(1):9-16.

Reid IR, Bolland MJ, Grey A. Effects of vitamin D supplements on bone mineral density: a systematic review and meta-analysis. Lancet. 2014 Jan 11;383(9912):146-55. doi: 10.1016/S0140-6736(13)61647-5.

Reilly T, Stevenson I. An investigation of the effects of negative air ions on responses to submaximal exercise at different times of day. *J Hum Ergol.* 1993 Jun;22(1):1-9.

Reiter RJ, Garcia JJ, Pie J. Oxidative toxicity in models of neurodegeneration: responses to melatonin. *Restor Neurol Neurosci.* 1998 Jun;12(2-3):135-42.

Reiter RJ, Tan DX, Korkmaz A, Erren TC, Piekarski C, Tamura H, Manchester LC. Light at night, chrono-disruption, melatonin suppression, and cancer risk: a review. *Crit Rev Oncog.* 2007;13(4):303-28.

Reiter RJ, Tan DX, Manchester LC, Qi W. Biochemical reactivity of melatonin with reactive oxygen and nitrogen species: a review of the evidence. *Cell Biochem Biophys.* 2001;34(2):237-56.

Roberts JE. Light and immunomodulation. *Ann N Y Acad Sci.* 2000;917:435-45.

Robinson TN. Television viewing and childhood obesity. *Pediatr Clin North Am.* 2001 Aug;48(4):1017-25.

Rodermel SR, Smith-Sonneborn J. Age-correlated changes in expression of micronuclear damage and repair in Paramecium tetraurelia. *Genetics.* 1977 Oct;87(2):259-74.

Rodriguez E, Valbuena MC, Rey M, Porras de Quintana L. Causal agents of photoallergic contact dermatitis diagnosed in the national institute of dermatology of Colombia. *Photodermatol Photoimmunol Photomed.* 2006 Aug;22(4):189-92.

Rollier A. *Le Pansement Solaire.* Paris: Payot, 1916.

Rosenthal N, Blehar M. *Seasonal affective disorders and phototherapy.* New York: Guildford Press, 1989.

Rossouw JE, Prentice RL, Manson JE, Wu L, Barad D, Barnabei VM, Ko M, LaCroix AZ, Margolis KL, Stefanick ML. Postmenopausal hormone therapy and risk of cardiovascular disease by age and years since menopause. *JAMA.* 2007 Apr 4;297(13):1465-77.

Rostand SG. Ultraviolet light may contribute to geographic and racial blood pressure differences. *Hypertension.* 1997 Aug;30(2 Pt 1):150-6.

Roy M, Kirschbaum C, Steptoe A. Intraindividual variation in recent stress exposure as a moderator of cortisol and testosterone levels. Ann Behav Med. 2003 Dec;26(3):194-200.

Royal Society of Canada *A Review of the Potential Health Risks of Radiofrequency Fields from Wireless Telecommunication Devices.* Ottawa: Royal Society of Canada. 1999.

Roybal K, Theobold D, Graham A, DiNieri JA, Russo SJ, Krishnan V, Chakravarty S, Peevey J, Oehrlein N, Birnbaum S, Vitaterna MH, Orsulak P, Takahashi JS, Nestler EJ, Carlezon WA Jr, McClung CA. Mania-like behavior induced by disruption of CLOCK. *Proc Natl Acad Sci USA* 2007;104(15):6406-6411.

Rubin E., Farber JL. *Pathology.* 3rd Ed. Philadelphia: Lippincott-Raven, 1999.

Rubin GJ, Hahn G, Everitt BS, Cleare AJ, Wessely S. Are some people sensitive to mobile phone signals? Within participants double blind randomised provocation study. *BMJ.* 2006 Apr 15;332(7546):886-91.

Russo PA, Halliday GM. Inhibition of nitric oxide and reactive oxygen species production improves the ability of a sunscreen to protect from sunburn, immunosuppression and photocarcinogenesis. *Br J Dermatol.* 2006 Aug;155(2):408-15.

Saarijarvi S, Lauerma H, Helenius H, Saarilehto S. Seasonal affective disorders among rural Finns and Lapps. *Acta Psychiatr Scand.* 1999 Feb;99(2):95-101.

Sahar S, Sassone-Corsi P. Circadian clock and breast cancer: a molecular link. *Cell Cycle.* 2007 Jun 1;6(11):1329-31.

Salama OE, Naga RM. Cellular phones: are they detrimental? *J Egypt Pub Hlth.* 2004;79(3-4):197-223.

Salford LG, Brun AE, Eberhardt JL, Malmgren L, Persson BR. Nerve cell damage in mammalian brain after exposure to microwaves from GSM mobile phones. *Environ Health Perspect.* 2003 Jun;111(7):881-3; discussion A408.

Sanders R. Slow brain waves play key role in coordinating complex activity. UC Berkeley News. 2006 Sep 14.

Sarveiya V, Risk S, Benson HA. Liquid chromatographic assay for common sunscreen agents: application to in vivo assessment of skin penetration and systemic absorption in human volunteers. *J Chromatogr B Analyt Technol Biomed Life Sci.* 2004 Apr 25;803(2):225-31.

Sato TK, Yamada RG, Ukai H, Baggs JE, Miraglia LJ, Kobayashi TJ, Welsh DK, Kay SA, Ueda HR, Hogenesch JB. Feedback repression is required for mammalian circadian clock function. *Nat Genet.* 2006 Mar;38(3):312-9.

Satyanarayana S, Sushruta K, Sarma GS, Srinivas N, Subba Raju GV. Antioxidant activity of the aqueous extracts of spicy food additives – evaluation and comparison with ascorbic acid in in-vitro systems. *J Herb Pharmacother.* 2004;4(2):1-10.

Savitz DA. Epidemiologic studies of electric and magnetic fields and cancer: strategies for extending knowledge. *Environ Health Perspect.* 1993 Dec;101 Suppl 4:83-91.

Schäfer A, Kratky KW. The effect of colored illumination on heart rate variability. *Forsch Komplementmed.* 2006 Jun;13(3):167-73.

Schirmacher A, Winters S, Fischer S, Goeke J, Galla HJ, Kullnick U, Ringelstein EB, Stögbauer F. Electromagnetic fields (1.8 GHz) increase the permeability to sucrose of the blood-brain barrier in vitro. *Bioelectromagnetics.* 2000 Jul;21(5):338-45.

Schlumpf M, Cotton B, Conscience M, Haller V, Steinmann B, Lichtensteiger W. In vitro and in vivo estrogenicity of UV screens. *Environ Health Perspect.* 2001 Mar;109(3):239-44.

Schmidt C, Collette F, Cajochen C, Peigneux P. A time to think: circadian rhythms in human cognition. *Cogn Neuropsychol.* 2007 Oct;24(7):755-89.

Schmitt B, Frölich L. Creative therapy options for patients with dementia – a systematic review. *Fortschr Neurol Psychiatr.* 2007 Dec;75(12):699-707.

Schreiber, G.H., Swaen, G.M., Meijers, J.M.M., Slangen, J.J.M., and Sturmans, F. Cancer mortality and residence near electricity transmission equipment: A retrospective cohort study. *Int. J. Epidemiol.* 1993;22:9–15.

Schulz TJ, Zarse K, Voigt A, Urban N, Birringer M, Ristow M. Glucose restriction extends Caenorhabditis elegans life span by inducing mitochondrial respiration and increasing oxidative stress. *Cell Metab.* 2007 Oct;6(4):280-93.

Schumacher P. *Biophysical Therapy Of Allergies.* Stuttgart: Thieme, 2005.

Schüz J, Mann S. A discussion of potential exposure metrics for use in epidemiological studies on human exposure to radiowaves from mobile phone base stations. *J Expo Anal Environ Epidemiol.* 2000 Nov-Dec;10(6 Pt 1):600-5.

Schwartz GG, Skinner HG. Vitamin D status and cancer: new insights. *Curr Opin Clin Nutr Metab Care.* 2007 Jan;10(1):6-11.

Schwartz S, De Mattei R, Brame E, Spottiswoode S. Infrared spectra alteration in water proximate to the palms of therapeutic practitioners. In: Wiener D, Nelson R (Eds.): *Research in parapsychology 1986.* Metuchen, NJ: Scarecrow Press, 1987:24-29.

Scott BO. The history of ultraviolet therapy. in Licht S. ed. *Therapeutic Electricity and Ultraviolet Radiation.* Phys Med Lib 4. Connecticut: Licht, 1967.

Serra-Valls A. Electromagnetic Industrion and the Conservation of Momentum in the Spiral Paradox. *Cornell University Library.* http://arxiv.org/ftp/physics/papers/0012/0012009.pdf. Accessed: 2007 July.

Shearman LP, Zylka MJ, Weaver DR, Kolakowski LF Jr, Reppert SM. Two period homologs: circadian expression and photic regulation in the suprachiasmatic nuclei. *Neuron.* 1997 Dec;19(6):1261-9.

Shevelev IA, Kostelianetz NB, Kamenkovich VM, Sharaev GA. EEG alpha-wave in the visual cortex: check of the hypothesis of the scanning process. *Int J Psychophysiol.* 1991 Aug;11(2):195-201.

Shivers RR, Kavaliers M, Teskey GC, Prato FS, Pelletier RM. Magnetic resonance imaging temporarily alters blood-brain barrier permeability in the rat. *Neurosci Lett.* 1987 Apr 23;76(1):25-31.

Sies H, Stahl W. Nutritional protection against skin damage from sunlight. Annu Rev Nutr. 2004;24:173-200.

Sita-Lumsden A, Lapthorn G, Swaminathan R, Milburn HJ. Reactivation of tuberculosis and vitamin D deficiency: the contribution of diet and exposure to sunlight. *Thorax.* 2007 Nov;62(11):1003-7.

Skwerer RG, Jacobsen FM, Duncan CC, Kelly KA, Sack DA, Tamarkin L, Gaist PA, Kasper S, Rosenthal NE. Neurobiology of Seasonal Affective Disorder and Phototherapy. *J Biolog Rhyth.* 1988;3(2):135-154.

Smith CW. Coherence in living biological systems. *Neural Network World.* 1994:4(3):379-388.

Smith MJ. Effect of Magnetic Fields on Enzyme Reactivity. In Barnothy M.(ed.), *Biological Effects of Magnetic Fields.* New York: Plenum Press, 1969.

Smith MJ. *The Influence on Enzyme Growth By the 'Laying on of Hands: Dimensions of Healing.* Los Altos, California: Academy of Parapsychology and Medicine, 1973.

Smith-Sonneborn J. Age-correlated effects of caffeine on non-irradiated and UV-irradiated Paramecium Aurelia. *J Gerontol.* 1974 May;29(3):256-60.

Smith-Sonneborn J. DNA repair and longevity assurance in Paramecium tetraurelia. *Science.* 1979 Mar 16;(4385):1115-7.

Smits MG, Williams A, Skene DJ, Von Schantz M. The 3111 Clock gene polymorphism is not associated with sleep and circadian rhythmicity in phenotypically characterized human subjects. *J Sleep Res.* 2002 Dec;11(4):305-12.

Snow WB. *The Therapeutics of Radiant Light and Heat and Convective Heat.* NY: Sci Auth Publ, 1909.

Snyder K. Researchers Produce Firsts with Bursts of Light: Team generates most energetic terahertz pulses yet, observes useful optical phenomena. *Press Release: Brookhaven National Laboratory.* 2007 July 24.

Soler M, Chandra S, Ruiz D, Davidson E, Hendrickson D, Christou G. A third isolated oxidation state for the Mn12 family of singl molecule magnets. *ChemComm;* 2000; Nov 22.

Spanagel R, Rosenwasser AM, Schumann G, Sarkar DK. Alcohol consumption and the body's biological clock. *Alcohol Clin Exp Res.* 2005 Aug;29(8):1550-7.

Speed Of Light May Not Be Constant, Physicist Suggests. *Science Daily.* 1999 Oct 6. www.sciencedaily.com/releases/1999/10/991005114024.htm. Accessed: 2007 June.

Spencer FA, Goldberg RJ, Becker RC, Gore JM. Seasonal distribution of acute myocardial infarction in the second National Registry of Myocardial Infarction. J Am Coll Cardiol. 1998 May;31(6):1226-33.

St Hilaire MA, Gronfier C, Zeitzer JM, Klerman EB. A physiologically based mathematical model of melatonin including ocular light suppression and interactions with the circadian pacemaker. *J Pineal Res.* 2007 Oct;43(3):294-304.

Stahl W, Heinrich U, Wiseman S, Eichler O, Sies H, Tronnier H. Dietary tomato paste protects against ultraviolet light-induced erythema in humans. *J Nutr.* 2001 May;131(5):1449-51.

Staples JA, Ponsonby AL, Lim LL, McMichael AJ. Ecologic analysis of some immune-related disorders, including type 1 diabetes, in Australia: latitude, regional ultraviolet radiation, and disease prevalence. *Environ Health Perspect.* 2003 Apr;111(4):518-23.

Steck B. Effects of optical radiation on man. *Light Resch Techn.* 1982;14:130-141.

Stephenson R. Circadian rhythms and sleep-related breathing disorders. *Sleep Med.* 2007 Sep;8(6):681-7.

Stoebner-Delbarre A, Thezenas S, Kuntz C, Nguyen C, Giordanella JP, Sancho-Garnier H, Guillot B; Le Groupe EPI-CES. Sun exposure and sun protection behavior and attitudes among the French population. *Ann Dermatol Venereol.* 2005 Aug-Sep;132(8-9 Pt 1):652-7.

Stoupel E, Babayev E, Mustafa F, Abramson E, Israelevich P, Sulkes J. Acute myocardial infarction occurrence: environmental links - Baku 2003-2005 data. *Med Sci Monit.* 2007 Aug;13(8):BR175-9.

Stoupel E, Monselise Y, Lahav J. Changes in autoimmune markers of the anti-cardiolipin syndrome on days of extreme geomagnetic activity. *J Basic Clin Physiol Pharmacol.* 2006;17(4):269-78.

Sugarman E. *Warning, The Electricity Around You May be Hazardous To Your Health.* NY: Sim & Schuster, 1992.

Sulman FG, Levy D, Lunkan L, Pfeifer Y, Tal E. New methods in the treatment of weather sensitivity. *Fortschr Med.* 1977 Mar 17;95(11):746-52.

Suppes P, Han B, Epelboim J, Lu ZL. Invariance of brain-wave representations of simple visual images and their names. *Proceedings of the National Academy of Sciences Psychology-BS.* 1999;96(25):14658-14663.

Swislocki A, Orth M, Bales M, Weisshaupt J, West C, Edrington J, Cooper B, Saputo L, Islas M, Miaskowski C. A randomized clinical trial of the effectiveness of photon stimulation on pain, sensation, and quality of life in patients with diabetic peripheral neuropathy. *J Pain Symptom Manage.* 2010 Jan;39(1):88-99. Epub 2009 Nov 5.

Tahvanainen K, Nino J, Halonen P, Kuusela T, Alanko T, Laitinen T, Lansimies E, Hietanen M, Lindholm H. Effects of cellular phone use on ear canal temperature measured by NTC thermistors. *Clin Physiol Funct Imaging.* 2007 May;27(3):162-72.

Tan DX, Manchester LC, Reiter RJ, Qi WB, Karbownik M, Calvo JR. Significance of melatonin in antioxidative defense system: reactions and products. *Biol Signals Recept.* 2000 May-Aug;9(3-4):137-59.

Taoka S, Padmakumar R, Grissom C, Banerjee R. Magnetic Field Effects on Coenzyme B-12 Dependent Enzymes: Validation of Ethanolamine Ammonia Lyase Results and Extension to Human Methylmalonyl CoA Mutase. *Bioelectromagnetics.* 1997;18: 506-513.

Taraban M, Leshina T, Anderson M, Grissom C. Magnetic Field Dependence and the Role of electron spin in Heme Enzymes: Horseradish Peroxidase. *J. Am. Chem. Soc.* 1997;119: 5768-5769.

Taskinen H, Kyyrönen P, Hemminki K. Effects of ultrasound, shortwaves, and physical exertion on pregnancy outcome in physiotherapists. *J Epidemiol Community Health.* 1990 Sep;44(3):196-201.

Tevini M, ed. *UV-B Radiation and Ozone Depletion: Effects on humans, animals, plants, microorganisms and materials.* Boca Raton: Lewis Pub, 1993.

Thaker JP, Patel MB, Jongnarangsin K, Liepa VV, Thakur RK. Electromagnetic interference with pacemakers caused by portable media players. *Heart Rhythm.* 2008 Apr;5(4):538-44.

Thakkar RR, Garrison MM, Christakis DA. A systematic review for the effects of television viewing by infants and preschoolers. *Pediatrics.* 2006 Nov;118(5):2025-31.

Thakur CP, Sharma D. Full moon and crime. *Br Med J.* 1984 December 22; 289(6460): 1789-1791.

Thomas MK, Lloyd-Jones DM, Thadhani RI, Shaw AC, Deraska DJ, Finkelstein JS, *et al.* Hypovitaminosis D in Medical Inpatients. *NEJM.* 1998 March 19;338(12):777-783.

Thompson D. *On Growth and Form.* Cambridge: Cambridge University Press, 1992.

Timofeev I, Steriade M. Low-frequency rhythms in the thalamus of intact-cortex and decorticated cats. *J Neurophysiol.* 1996 Dec;76(6):4152-68.

Ting W, Schultz K, Cac NN, Peterson M, Walling HW. Tanning bed exposure increases the risk of malignant melanoma. *Int J Dermatol.* 2007 Dec;46(12):1253-7.

Tiwari M. *Ayurveda: A Life of Balance.* Rochester, VT: Healing Arts, 1995.

Tomasek L, Rogel A, Tirmarche M, Mitton N, Laurier D. Lung cancer in French and Czech uranium miners: Radon-associated risk at low exposure rates and modifying effects of time since exposure and age at exposure. *Radiat Res.* 2008 Feb;169(2):125-37.

Tomasek L, Rogel A, Tirmarche M, Mitton N, Laurier D. Lung cancer in French and Czech uranium miners: Radon-associated risk at low exposure rates and modifying effects of time since exposure and age at exposure. *Radiat Res.* 2008 Feb;169(2):125-37.

Toomer G. "Ptolemy". *The Dictionary of Scientific Biography.* New York: Gale Cengage, 1970.

Tripkovic L, Lambert H, Hart K, Smith CP, Bucca G, Penson S, Chope G, Hyppönen E, Berry J, Vieth R, Lanham-New S. Comparison of vitamin D2 and vitamin D3 supplementation in raising serum 25-

hydroxyvitamin D status: a systematic review and meta-analysis. Am J Clin Nutr. 2012 Jun;95(6):1357-64. doi: 10.3945/ajcn.111.031070.

Tsinkalovsky O, Smaaland R, Rosenlund B, Sothern RB, Hirt A, Steine S, Badiee A, Abrahamsen JF, Eiken HG, Laerum OD. Circadian variations in clock gene expression of human bone marrow CD34+ cells. *J Biol Rhythms.* 2007 Apr;22(2):140-50.

Tsong T. Deciphering the language of cells. *Trends in Biochem Sci.* 1989;14: 89-92.

Tweed K. Study: Conceiving in Summer Lowers Baby's Future Test Scores. *Fox News.* 2007 May 9, 2007. (Study done by: Winchester P. 2007. Pediatric Academic Societies annual meeting.)

Ulrich RS. Aesthetic and affective response to natural environment. In Altman, I. and Wohlwill, J. F. (eds) *Human Behaviour and Environment: Advances in Theory and Research. Volume 6: Behaviour and the Natural Environment.* New York: Plenum Press: 1983:85-125.

Ulrich RS. Influences of passive experiences with plants on individual wellbeing and health. In Relf, D. (ed) *The Role of Horticulture in Human Well-Being and Social Development: A National Symposium.* Portland: Timber Press, Portland. 1992:93 -105.

Ulrich RS. Natural versus urban scenes: some psychophysiological effects. *Environment and Behaviour.* 1981:523-556.

Ulrich RS. View through window may influence recovery from surgery. *Science.* 1984;224:420 - 421.

Ulrich RS. Visual landscapes and psychological well being. *Landscape Research.* 1979;4:17-23.

Van Cauter E. Slow wave sleep and release of growth hormone. *JAMA.* 2000 Dec 6;284(21):2717-8.

Vaquero JM, Gallego MC. Sunspot numbers can detect pandemic influenza A: the use of different sunspot numbers. *Med Hypotheses.* 2007;68(5):1189-90.

Vena JE, Graham S, Hellmann R, Swanson M, Brasure J. Use of electric blankets and risk of postmenopausal breast cancer. *Am J Epidemiol.* 1991 Jul 15;134(2):180-5.

Vgontzas AN. The diagnosis and treatment of chronic insomnia in adults. *Sleep.* 2005 Sep 1;28(9):1047-8.

Villani S. Impact of media on children and adolescents: a 10-year review of the research. *J Am Acad Child Adolesc Psychiatry.* 2001 Apr;40(4):392-401.

Viner RM, Cole TJ. Television viewing in early childhood predicts adult body mass index. *J Pediatr.* 2005 Oct;147(4):429-35.

Viola AU, James LM, Schlangen LJ, Dijk DJ. Blue-enriched white light in the workplace improves self-reported alertness, performance and sleep quality. *Scand J Work Environ Hlth.* 2008 Aug;34(4):297-306.

von Schantz M, Archer SN. Clocks, genes and sleep. *J R Soc Med.* 2003 Oct;96(10):486-9.

Walch JM, Rabin BS, Day R, Williams JN, Choi K, Kang JD. The effect of sunlight on postoperative analgesic medication use: a prospective study of patients undergoing spinal surgery. *Psychosom Med.* 2005 Jan-Feb;67(1):156-63.

Walker M. *The Power of Color.* New Delhi: B. Jain Publishers. 2002.

Watson L. *Beyond Supernature.* New York: Bantam, 1987.

Wayne R. *Chemistry of the Atmospheres.* Oxford Press, 1991.

Weaver J, Astumian R. The response of living cells to very weak electric fields: the thermal noise limit. *Science.* 1990;247: 459-462.

Weller A, Weller L. Menstrual synchrony between mothers and daughters and between roommates. *Physiol Behav.* 1993 May;53(5):943-9.

Weller L, Weller A, Roizman S. Human menstrual synchrony in families and among close friends: examining the importance of mutual exposure. *J Comp Psychol.* 1999 Sep;113(3):261-8.

Welsh D, Yoo SH, Liu A, Takahashi J, Kay S. Bioluminescence Imaging of Individual Fibroblasts Reveals Persistent, Independently Phased Circadian Rhythms of Clock Gene Expression. *Current Biology.* 2004;14:2289-2295.

Wertheimer N, Leeper E. Electrical wiring configurations and childhood cancer. *Am J Epidemiol.* 1979 Mar;109(3):273-84.

West P. *Surf Your Biowaves.* London: Quantum, 1999.

Weyandt TB, Schrader SM, Turner TW, Simon SD. Semen analysis of military personnel associated with military duty assignments. *Reprod Toxicol.* 1996 Nov-Dec;10(6):521-8.

Wharton B, Bishop N. Rickets. *Lancet.* 2003 Oct 25;362(9393):1389-400.

Whittaker E. *History of the Theories of Aether and Electricity.* New York: Nelson LTD, 1953.

Wilen J, Hornsten R, Sandstrom M, Bjerle P, Wiklund U, Stensson O, Lyskov E, Mild KH. Electromagnetic field exposure and health among RF plastic sealer operators. *Bioelectromag.* 2004 Jan;25(1):5-15.

Williams MC, Lecluyse K, Rock-Faucheux A. Effective interventions for reading disability. *J Am Optom Assoc.* 1992 Jun;63(6):411-7.

Winchester AM. *Biology and its Relation to Mankind.* New York: Van Nostrand Reinhold, 1969.

Winfree AT. *The Timing of Biological Clocks.* New York: Scientific American, 1987.

Winstead DK, Schwartz BD, Bertrand WE. Biorhythms: fact or superstition? *Am J Psychiatry.* 1981 Sep;138(9):1188-92.

Wolf, M. Beyond the Point Particle - *A Wave Structure for the Electron. Galil Electrodyn.* 1995 Oct;6(5):83-91.

Wolpowitz D, Gilchrest BA. The vitamin D questions: how much do you need and how should you get it? *J Am Acad Dermatol* 2006;54:301-17.

Wolverton BC. *How to Grow Fresh Air: 50 House Plants that Purify Your Home or Office.* NY: Penguin, 1997.

Wyart C, Webster WW, Chen JH, Wilson SR, McClary A, Khan RM, Sobel N. Smelling a single component of male sweat alters levels of cortisol in women. *J Neurosci.* 2007 Feb 7;27(6):1261-5.

Yamaoka Y. Solid cell nest (SCN) of the human thyroid gland. *Acta Pathol Jpn.* 1973 Aug;23(3):493-506.

Yeager RL, Oleske DA, Sanders RA, Watkins JB 3rd, Eells JT, Henshel DS. Melatonin as a principal component of red light therapy. *Med Hypotheses.* 2007;69(2):372-6.

Yeung JW. A hypothesis: Sunspot cycles may detect pandemic influenza A in 1700-2000 A.D. *Med Hypotheses.* 2006;67(5):1016-22.

Zaets VN, Karpov PA, Smertenko PS, Blium IaB. Molecular mechanisms of the repair of UV-induced DNA damages in plants. *Tsitol Genet.* 2006 Sep-Oct;40(5):40-68.

Zimmerman FJ, Christakis DA. Children's television viewing and cognitive outcomes: a longitudinal analysis of national data. *Arch Pediatr Adolesc Med.* 2005 Jul;159(7):619-25.

Zittermann A, Schleithoff SS, Koerfer R. Vitamin D insufficiency in congestive heart failure: why and what to do about it? *Heart Fail Rev.* 2006 Mar;11(1):25-33.

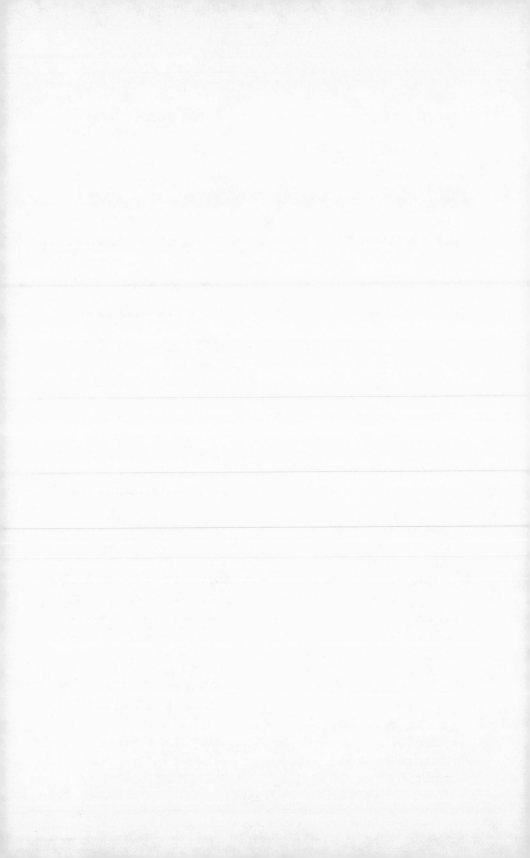

Index

magnets, 69, 73, 76
malanopsin, 20
mango, 182
mania, 19, 196
mechanical waves, 93
medium frequency (MF), 145
melanin, 193, 194, 195, 201,
  207, 209, 210, 211, 217, 218
melanocytes, 194, 195, 201,
  209, 217
melanoma, 136, 147, 151,
  200, 201, 202, 203, 207,
  209, 214
melanosomes, 195
melatonin, 17, 20, 22, 23, 25,
  26, 27, 28, 29, 35, 36, 39,
  50, 51, 53, 61, 62, 120, 144,
  155, 163, 164, 178, 179,
  184, 187, 192, 197, 198, 199
membrane polarization, 74
memory, 32, 33, 42, 45, 136,
  152, 156, 178, 185
menigioma, 151
menstruation, 47, 49, 50, 53
Merkel cell carcinoma, 202
mesosphere, 14
methyl-benzylidene camphor,
  206
micro-capillaries, 129, 130
microcirculation, 131
microwave rays, 14
mid-day sun, 63, 115, 117,
  130, 134, 183, 205
mid-wave infrared, 123
Milky Way, 15, 90, 101
minerals, 35, 108, 157, 213,
  221
minimal erythemal dose, 210

mood, 27, 45, 56, 112, 135,
  165, 181, 183, 184, 195,
  196, 197, 217
moon, 3, 4, 5, 6, 8, 11, 14, 25,
  47, 51, 52, 53, 54, 55, 63,
  77, 117, 168
morning, 11, 22, 28, 29, 30,
  31, 34, 39, 40, 47, 61, 62,
  63, 64, 116, 121, 126, 131,
  132, 179, 183, 187, 211,
  217, 218, 219
MP3 player, 154
multiple sclerosis, 68, 194,
  198
mustard, 182
myeloma, 200
myocardial infarction, 67, 193
natural fiber, 80, 81, 185
near infrared, 123
negotiation, 179, 185
nephrotoxins, 158
nervous diseases, 192
neuralgia, 191
neurotoxins, 158
neurotransmitters, 17, 18, 24,
  26, 34, 37, 38, 105, 184,
  192, 216, 217
non-Hodgkin's lymphoma,
  200
non-ionizing radiation, 137,
  138, 139, 165
norepinephrine, 192
North Pole, 72
nuclear electricity generating
  plant, 139
nuclear magnetic resonance,
  76
nuts, 62, 182, 204, 215